The Extended Meridians of Zen Shiatsu

of related interest

Shiatsu Theory and Practice
Carola Beresford-Cooke
ISBN 978 1 84819 308 6
eISBN 978 0 85701 260 9

Baby Shiatsu
Gentle Touch to Help your Baby Thrive
Karin Kalbantner-Wernicke and Tina Haase
Illustrated by Monika Werneke
ISBN 978 1 84819 104 4
eISBN 978 0 85701 086 5

The Extended Meridians of Zen Shiatsu

A Guidebook and Colouring Book

Elaine Liechti and Vicky Smyth
Foreword by Carola Beresford-Cooke
Photographs by David Boni

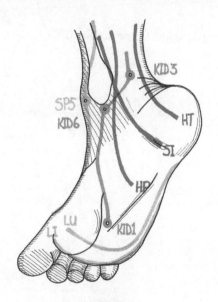

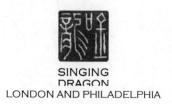

SINGING
DRAGON
LONDON AND PHILADELPHIA

First published in 2017
by Singing Dragon
an imprint of Jessica Kingsley Publishers
73 Collier Street
London N1 9BE, UK
and
400 Market Street, Suite 400
Philadelphia, PA 19106, USA

www.singingdragon.com

Library of Congress Cataloging in Publication Data
A CIP catalog record for this book is available from the Library of Congress

British Library Cataloguing in Publication Data
A CIP catalogue record for this book is available from the British Library

ISBN 978 1 84819 319 2

Printed and bound by CPI Group (UK) Ltd, Croydon, CR0 4YY

Dedicated to Oliver and Rosie, my finest teachers.

Vicky

Contents

Foreword

Although Shiatsu is sometimes described as 'acupuncture without needles', in practice it is nothing like acupuncture; the two are different branches of the same great tree of East Asian medicine. Acupuncture has been studied and documented for hundreds of years, and in tandem with the mounting volume of acupuncture theory and literature has grown the potential for its practice to become formulaic and theoretical. Shiatsu, however, is bodywork, and the practice of bodywork opens into a realm of fresh, vivid and immediate sensations that are difficult to express in writing and are consequently rarely documented.

For the 'giver', these sensations are a journey of exploration and understanding; for the 'receiver' they are a way of re-discovering and re-connecting with lost parts of him- or herself and thus of self-healing. For both, the process is relaxing, enlivening, uplifting and pleasurable.

And yet, notwithstanding its great potential, bodywork has been consistently undervalued as a therapy, perhaps partly because it is pleasurable, certainly in part because its practice is so little documented. No formula has been laid down for its wide-ranging action on mind as well as body; no vocabulary exists to express or interpret the rich and vivid world of experience it opens up to us.

Until comparatively recently, Shiatsu has similarly languished in obscurity as the poor relation of acupuncture; but the 1960s and '70s saw a ground-breaking milestone in its long history, with the publication, first in Japan and then in the West, of the work of Shizuto Masunaga. He interpreted the traditional theory in a new way, compatible with Western scientific understanding while remaining true to its roots in timeless Eastern philosophy. He also provided a method of practice that brought that philosophy into the physical dimension – Yin and Yang in action – with the experience of qualities that Shiatsu practitioners call *kyo* and *jitsu*. And, finally, he brought together the complex of meridian pathways (muscle meridians, connecting meridians, deep pathways, partners in the Six Divisions) into a comprehensive meridian system that can be followed throughout the body.

The Chinese word for the meridian system is *jingluo*, which includes the meanings of 'something woven', a 'network' or 'web'. An acupuncture classic states:

we should remember that the channel network is considerably more complex than…the superficial pathways of the twelve primary channels and there is no part of the body, no kind of tissue, no single cell, that is not supplied by the channels. (Deadman, Al-Khafaji and Baker 2007)

Masunaga's meridian system reflects this understanding of the meridian web that goes everywhere in the body and connects every part with every other part.

Masunaga's meridians, the 'extended' or 'Zen' meridians, supplement rather than replace the classical meridians of acupuncture. They include all the ancient versions as well as those mentioned above, and, with a little practice and training, they can be *felt*. Finding the meridians by touch is a part of Shiatsu training. In consequence, the Masunaga meridian chart is not a carefully measured map, like the Chinese acupuncture charts in which each point is immovably located; instead, it provides *guidance* about where the meridian is likely to be. This method of finding by touch is characteristically Japanese, and in Japanese acupuncture the points are found by feeling rather than by careful measuring. The Japanese understand what the Danish mathematician Tor Norretranders wrote, based on brain research findings: 'trust your hunches and intuitions – they are closer to reality than your perceived reality as they are based on far more information' (Norretranders 1999, p.272). They know that intuition gives us greater accuracy than measurement when we work with life forces; they are interested in the territory rather than the map.

Learning where the twelve extended pathways are *most likely* to be throughout the body is an essential part of Shiatsu training. Then, with practice, the true meridian can be found within that area of probability. Finding these flows sensitizes us to unfamiliar but thrilling sensations, leads us into a new way of experiencing the body. The meridians are the great advantage that distinguishes Shiatsu as a form of energy medicine. To ease the passage into learning them, Elaine Liechti and Vicky Smyth have produced a guidebook that is comprehensive and detailed, while allowing the student full freedom and encouragement to find the meridian flow by feel.

Elaine and I studied together with Pauline Sasaki, a former student of Masunaga and a Master of Shiatsu in her own right. Together we learned to turn the squiggles on Masunaga's meridian chart into recognizable pathways on the bodies of our fellow students. We also experienced the thrill of working directly with Ki via the meridians, an experience that previous, more formulaic approaches had not offered us. Elaine has brought this vital connection, together with her own wealth of experience from decades of Shiatsu practice and teaching, into the text of this wonderful book. Notes on helpful positions, tips for remembering the pathway in relation to the function it performs in the body and space for recording your own experiences and insights make this guidebook a unique teaching aid. Vicky's illustrations manage to combine clarity with beauty; one can almost feel the Ki flowing in her transparent meridian lines as they emerge from the background of muscles and bones. Photos clarify the best positions for treating the pathways. Among the several 'atlases' of the Shiatsu meridians, this is a uniquely comprehensive yet liberal and eclectic guidebook.

Shiatsu is only now beginning to recognize itself, both in its ancient history and its modern development. The task of amassing a Shiatsu literary tradition is only just beginning, and wise Shiatsu teachers are taking care to recognize and respect the differences between each others' approaches, in order to keep Shiatsu as an experience of our basic humanity and at the same time unique to each individual practitioner. This book is careful to maintain this open approach, which I hope will distinguish Shiatsu literature henceforth. Each teacher adds her own experience and interpretation to the authority, handed down by oral tradition, of the masters who have gone before, without claiming that hers is the only way. In this way Shiatsu is true to itself, enriches itself and hands those riches down to further generations of students of this powerful and profound healing practice.

Carola Beresford-Cooke, MRSS(T)

Acknowledgements

My biggest thanks go to Elaine, my first teacher, guide, inspirer, support and friend. This book is one of her many inspiring visions.

I am also grateful to Pauline Sasaki and Clifford Andrews for lighting the way; and Carola Beresford-Cooke and Paul Lundberg for their detailed accuracy and generous teaching of the location of meridians.

Thanks must also go to the many students of the Glasgow School of Shiatsu, from Silver to Rose groups, who have worked patiently with the evolving diagrams and whose feedback has been invaluable.

Vicky Smyth

My deepest thanks are to my main teacher and inspiration, Pauline Sasaki. It was Pauline who taught me Masunaga's extended meridian system and guided my Shiatsu development over many years. I also have to thank many classes of students at the Glasgow School of Shiatsu, who asked for clarification of locations so often that Vicky was inspired to make these drawings. It has taken a long time to bring this project to fruition, but we hope that the format of this book will be of assistance to both present and future students and practitioners of Shiatsu.

Elaine Liechti

About the Book

Like many Shiatsu students and teachers, we learnt the extended Zen Shiatsu meridians by listening to and watching our teacher – in our case Pauline Sasaki.

Masunaga's meridian map was an often-consulted reference to remind us of location outside of class and away from our teacher's expertise. However, when we came to teach these 'supplementary/extended meridians' we found that the very complexity of the map, with all the meridians drawn onto one figure, made it a less than ideal teaching aid. There also seemed to be anomalies between the front and side views, which made it difficult to follow the flow of the meridians in some cases between the neck and shoulders. We decided to draw out each meridian individually in a fairly precise anatomical way in order to make the pathways clearer to our students. Gathering all the drawings together in book form developed as an idea several years after the drawings had initially been completed.

There are inevitably difficulties in representing the three dimensions of the human body in a two-dimensional medium (i.e. on a flat page). Despite these difficulties our students at the Glasgow School of Shiatsu have found these diagrams a useful learning aid, and we hope they will help you too.

The illustrations presented here are the result of quite a number of years of drawing, re-drawing, discussing and much palpating for 'Where exactly does it go?' Of course, like all meridian charts 'the map is not the terrain' – you have to *feel* the meridian pathway for yourself. Masunaga himself said 'meridian widths are variable and sometimes their pathways change and are varied…' (Masunaga 1970, p.6). So this book is not intended by any means to be a definitive version of where the extended meridians run: it is where we find them in our practice. Just as a guidebook describes the major features of a city, but is not the city itself, we hope this book will be a route map to guide you to accurate location while you are learning to feel the extended meridians for yourself. Let the Fire of your intuition and feeling temper the Metallic need to 'get the location right'!

How to Use this Book

This book is designed to be your meridian notebook, where you can write notes and colour the diagrams and pictures in order to personalize how you learn the locations.

To enable you to get the most from the book we have set it out as a workbook. Each meridian view has a text page alongside with our comments plus space for you to write your own notes. The lines of the meridians are in an open format so that you can colour them in; you might choose the traditional shades of red for Fire meridians and green for Wood, or whatever colours appeal to you. Once you have coloured in a page, or even a whole meridian, you might want to consult the Colour Meridian Charts towards the end of the book to see where the meridian you have just coloured fits in relation to the other meridians.

We have included photos where a written description of a particular treatment position might not give sufficient detail. We suggest that you draw the meridians onto the photos to help make the locations more real to you. Within each section you will find our comments including favourite treatment positions, reminders about traditional meridian pathways and indications of point location in relation to the extended meridians. Over the years we have found that visual imagery has helped our students to gain greater clarity in regard to meridian location, so we have included this too, to help you with feeling and memorizing.

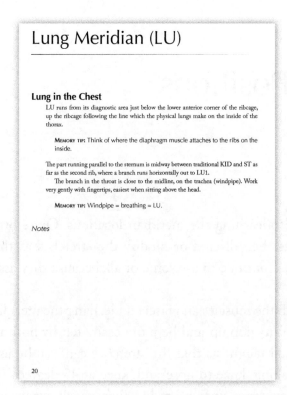

Lung Meridian (LU)

Lung in the Chest

LU runs from its diagnostic area just below the lower anterior corner of the ribcage, up the ribcage following the line which the physical lungs make on the inside of the thorax.

MEMORY TIP: Think of where the diaphragm muscle attaches to the ribs on the inside.

The part running parallel to the sternum is midway between traditional KID and ST as far as the second rib, where a branch runs horizontally out to LU1.

The branch in the throat is close to the midline, on the trachea (windpipe). Work very gently with fingertips, easiest when sitting above the head.

MEMORY TIP: Windpipe = breathing = LU.

Notes

20

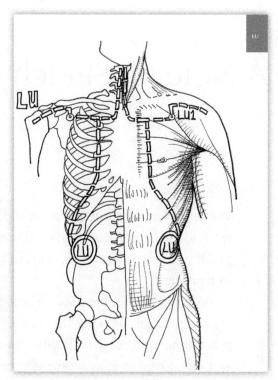

The meridians illustrated in this book are only the extended ones: the traditional meridians are so well-documented that we see no need to create further illustrations for them. However, in some cases we have shown part of the traditional pathway where it joins the extended system. The definitive text which we use at the Glasgow School of Shiatsu for traditional meridian location is *Essentials of Chinese Acupuncture* (Beijing College of Traditional Medicine 1980).

As an additional aid to study we have included Masunaga's diagnostic areas and Bo points, the names of major muscles, plus some beginning/ending acupoints. If anatomy is not your strong point then we recommend that in conjunction with this book you use an anatomy book such as *The Concise Book of Muscles* (Jarmey 2015).

We hope that you will find this interactive format useful in exploring the extended meridian system. Learning the meridian extensions can seem daunting, but the benefits of eventually being able to access all twelve meridians in all parts of the body make the task of learning them well worthwhile. If using this book can make that task more meaningful and personal then we shall have achieved our aim in creating it.

A Note on Stretch Positions

We teach stretch positions as an aid to learning the meridian locations. Quite often we find that once learnt, practitioners then discard or modify the stretches as their practice develops. However, some of us continue to use some or all, because they assist in treatment.

When placed in the relevant stretch the muscles and fascia underlying the meridian are accentuated, allowing the meridian to 'pop up' and be more easily felt by both the practitioner and receiver. Pauline Sasaki taught us that the stretches can also be used as a diagnostic tool: in supine if stretching 'knee to nose' and 'knee at 45 degrees' feel comfortable, but 'knee to opposite shoulder' is uncomfortable, then check out what is 'going on' in the KID meridian.

The list below details the most commonly used stretches as we were taught them by Pauline: some have been mentioned within the text and illustrated with photos, some are self-evident, some are illustrated here for clarity.

Arm stretches supine
(Working round the arm from Yin to Yang)

LU (trad.) and SP (Zen): arm at 4 o'clock/8 o'clock – see photo on page 42

HP (trad.): arm at 3 o'clock/9 o'clock

LIV (Zen): arm at 2 o'clock/10 o'clock – see photo on page 94

HT (trad.): arm above head and bent at elbow

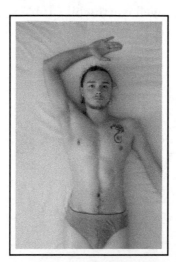

KID (Zen): shake hands position – see photo on page 62

SI (trad.): arm bent at elbow across chest

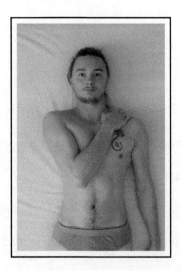

ST (Zen) and TH (trad.): arm in sling position – see photo on page 36

GB (Zen) and LI (trad.): 4 o'clock/8 o'clock posterior surface uppermost

BL (Zen): shake hands position – see photo on page 62

Leg stretches supine
(Working round the leg in a rotation)

SP (trad.): toe to ankle

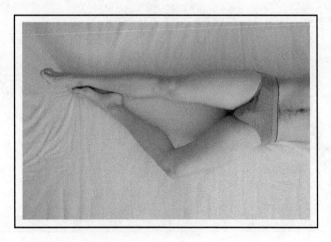

SI (Zen): heel to knee – see photo on page 54

HP (Zen): instep to knee – see photo on page 76

LIV (trad.): toe to knee

KID (trad.): as LIV but with lower leg open to allow access to KID10

HT (Zen): ankle over thigh (in practice we never use this but treat HT in prone – see page 46)

BL (trad.): knee to same side shoulder

LU (Zen): knee to nose

KID (Zen): knee to opposite shoulder – see photo on page 68

LI (Zen): knee at 45 degrees, push away – see photo on page 26

GB (trad.): instep to knee, push away

TH (Zen): toe to ankle, push away – see photo on page 82

ST (trad.): leg straight, plantar flex foot (or, if the receiver is very flexible, ankle to buttock)

On the photo below you can mark in the sequence (medial to lateral) HT, BL, LU, KID, LI.

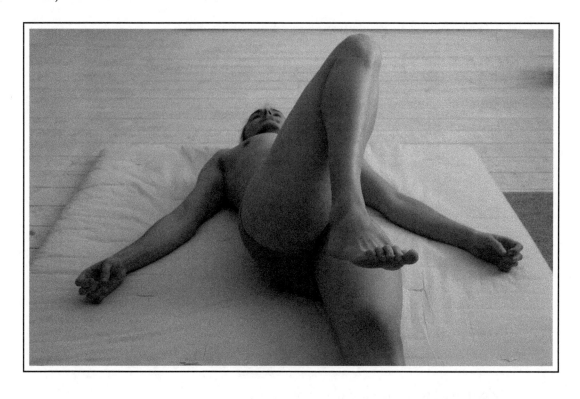

In preparing this manuscript Elaine realized she has been teaching and using the leg supine stretches SP, SI, HP and LIV at one position lower than most teachers; that is, SP – instep to ankle, SI – toe to ankle, HP – heel to knee, LIV – instep to knee. This works for her and for many students; however, the positions detailed in the text and lists above are those most commonly used by Zen Shiatsu teachers.

Leg stretches prone
(Only those meridians easily accessible and normally worked in prone)

HT (Zen): leg straight, work on medial aspect of opposite leg – see page 46

BL (trad.): leg straight

LU (Zen): leg straight

KID (Zen and trad.): leg straight for thigh, lift and abduct ankle for trad. in lower leg

LI (Zen): foot tucked over opposite ankle – see photo on page 28

GB (trad.): knee abducted to 90 degrees to the body and lower leg positioned 90 degrees to the thigh, 'like steps'

TH (Zen) and ST (trad.) are sometimes described as accessible in prone but we find it is much more effective to work them in side and supine respectively.

Lung Meridian (LU)

Lung in the Chest

LU runs from its diagnostic area just below the lower anterior corner of the ribcage, up the ribcage following the line which the physical lungs make on the inside of the thorax.

> **Memory tip:** Think of where the diaphragm muscle attaches to the ribs on the inside.

The part running parallel to the sternum is midway between traditional KID and ST as far as the second rib, where a branch runs horizontally out to LU1.

The branch in the throat is close to the midline, on the trachea (windpipe). Work very gently with fingertips, easiest when sitting above the head.

> **Memory tip:** Windpipe = breathing = LU.

Notes

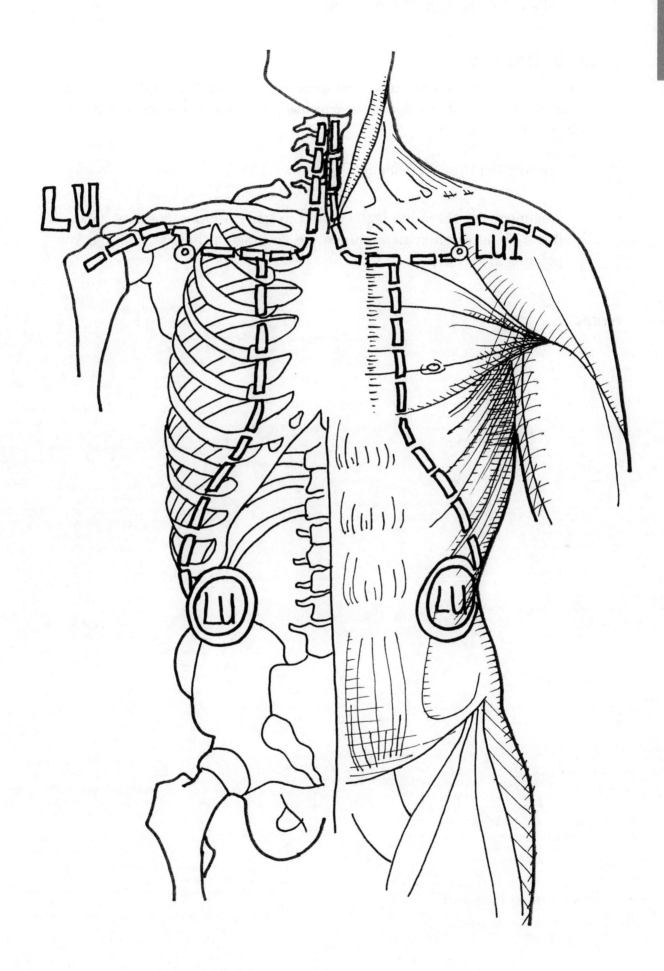

Lung in the Leg

LU in the leg runs directly parallel and lateral to traditional BL. At the foot it curls under the sole to end in a line at the proximal part of the ball of the foot. See also Colour Meridian Chart 14.

Memory tip: Nose = breathing = LU.

Treatment tip: LU in the leg is easiest to treat in prone position, although it can be accessed in supine using the 'leverage technique' with the knee pointing to the nose.

Notes

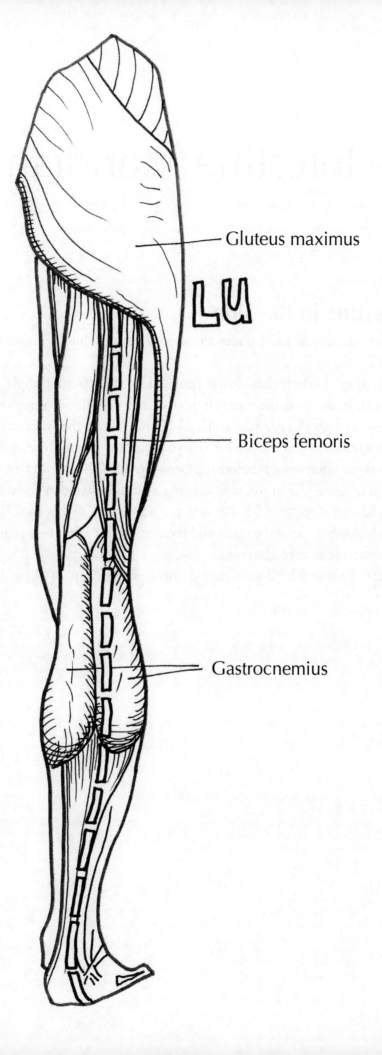

Gluteus maximus

LU

Biceps femoris

Gastrocnemius

Large Intestine Meridian (LI)

Large Intestine in the Side

Traditional LI ends at LI20 under the *opposite* nostril, but is illustrated here on the same side for clarity.

In the sides LI branches down from LI15 (the 'front dimple' when the arm is abducted), runs down the anterior part of the side (if we imagine the body as a 'cornflakes box' with a front, sides and back, LI runs down the anterior edge of the box), then snakes backwards at the waist to curve round the greater trochanter.

There is an interesting relationship between LI, GB and TH in arms, sides and legs. If you imagine GB in the side as being a straight wooden wand (see page 85 for location), LI runs directly in front of it to the waist, then snakes back. TH runs directly to the back of GB as far as the waist and then snakes forwards (see page 78), rather like the Caduceus, the staff of Hermes.

See also Colour Meridian Chart 6 for a comparison of these three meridians' location.

Notes

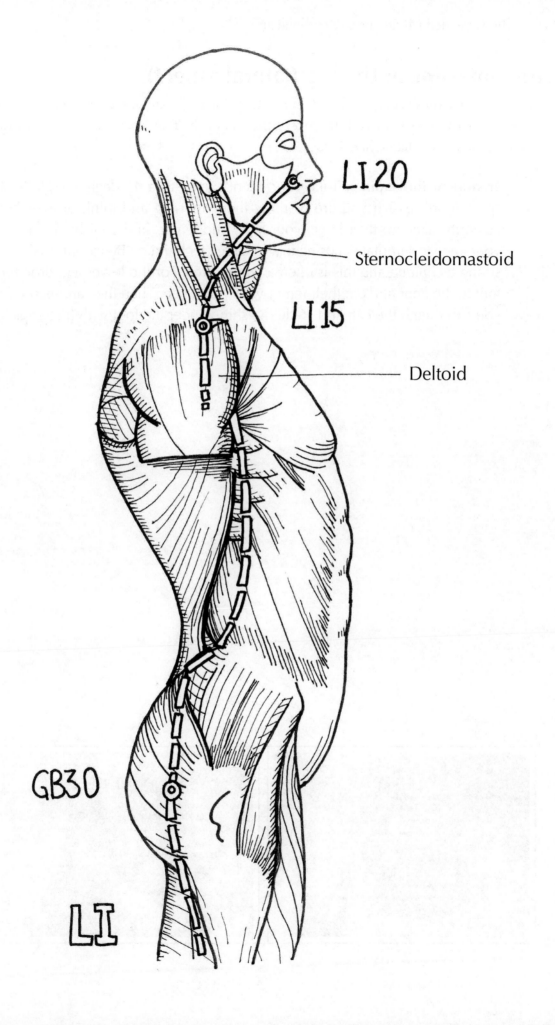

LI 20

Sternocleidomastoid

LI 15

Deltoid

GB30

LI

Large Intestine in the Leg (lateral aspect)

LI in the leg runs parallel and posterior to traditional GB and then curls under the sole of the foot to finish at the distal part of the ball of the foot, near the roots of the toes (see Colour Meridian Chart 14).

> **Treatment tip (supine):** Take your client's knee to a 45-degree angle to the spine (north east if you are working their right leg and think of their head as north). Line up their knee, your knee and femur, and your hara, then use your knee to stimulate LI using the 'leverage technique'. Be careful as this is a strong technique and this is often a tender area. For the lower leg, drop their foot to the floor and pin their femur with your knee. Then they are secure and you can thumb the calf and ankle, finishing under the foot with fingertips.

Notes

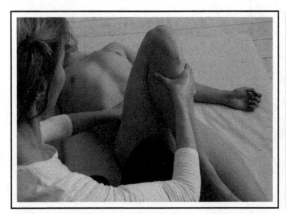 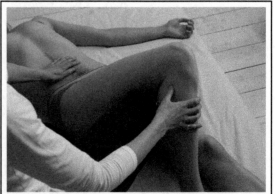

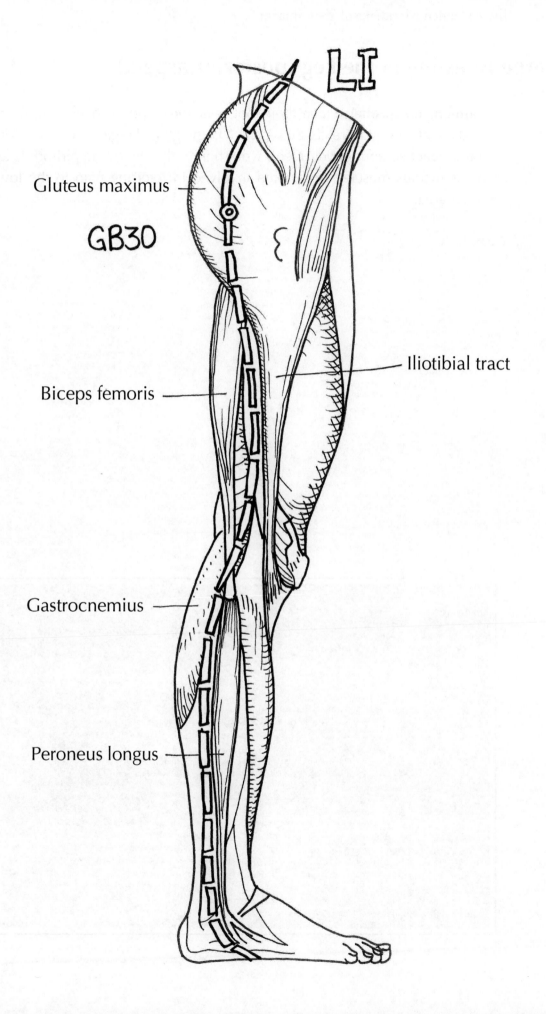

LI

Gluteus maximus

GB30

Biceps femoris

Iliotibial tract

Gastrocnemius

Peroneus longus

Large Intestine in the Leg (posterior aspect)

Treatment tip (prone): Place their foot over the opposite heel to bring the meridian into a slight stretch. Be sensitive in the gluteal region as the meridian is often reactive and tender. Deep work here will release the piriformis and gluteus medius muscles, both often involved in referring pain to the lower lumbar area.

Notes

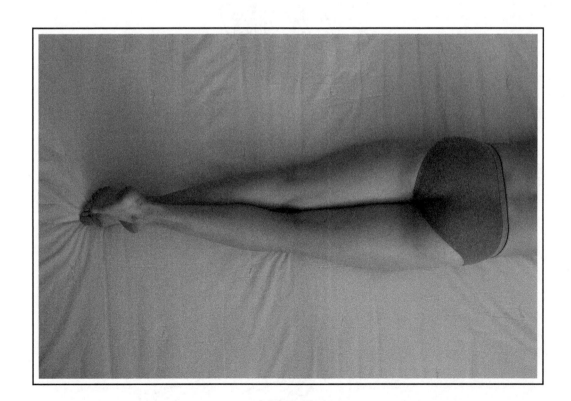

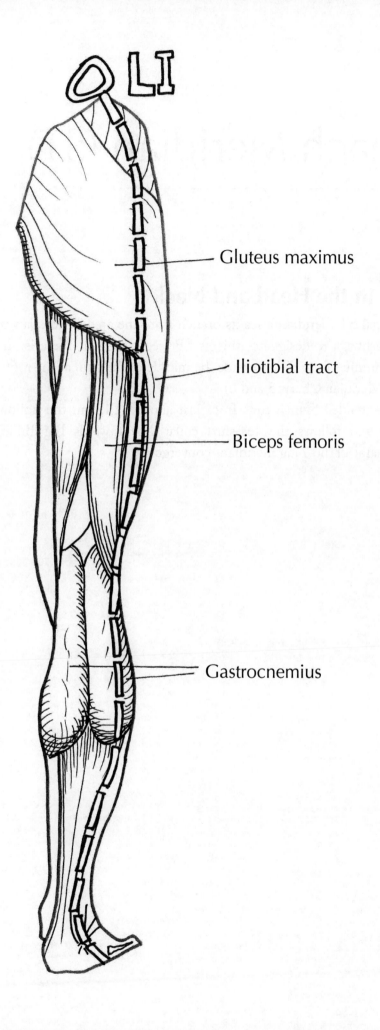

LI

Gluteus maximus

Iliotibial tract

Biceps femoris

Gastrocnemius

Stomach Meridian (ST)

Stomach in the Head and Neck

Traditional ST meridian loses its branch from the angle of the jaw up the side of the face: Masunaga re-designates this as SP (see page 38). There is an additional small branch running from ST6 towards the middle of the chin at the roots of the teeth (see Colour Meridian Charts 5 and 6).

The extended branch runs from just above ST12 (in the hollow superior to the clavicle) and follows the 'tee-shirt collar' line towards Big Bone (GV14), where traditionally all the Yang meridians converge.

Notes

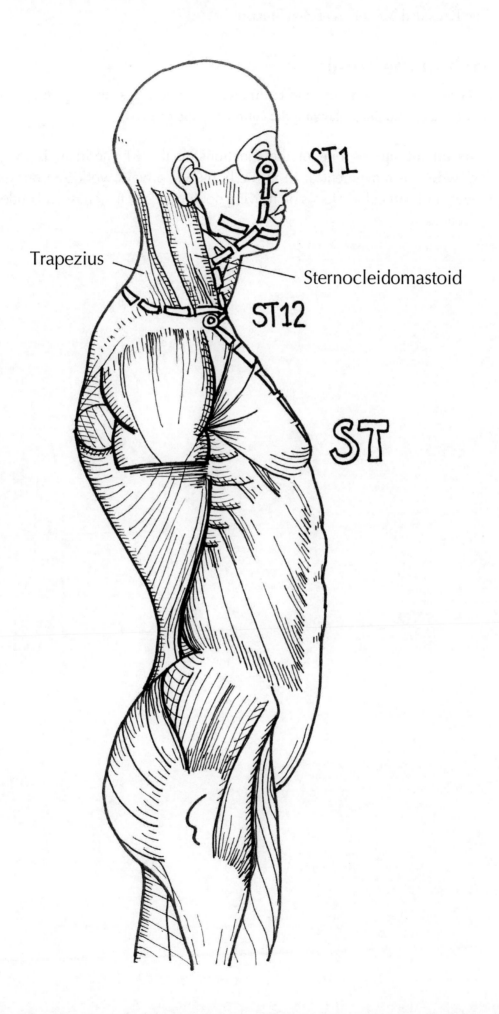

ST1

Trapezius

Sternocleidomastoid

ST12

ST

ST

Stomach in the Trunk

ST in the chest is the same as in traditional meridian maps, although the Masunaga chart has a curved line, following the contour of the chest.

> **Treatment tip:** As one of the functions of the ST meridian is to govern downwards movement of Ki in the body, we always work ST from head to feet, and particularly focus on moving downwards in the chest and abdominal area.

Notes

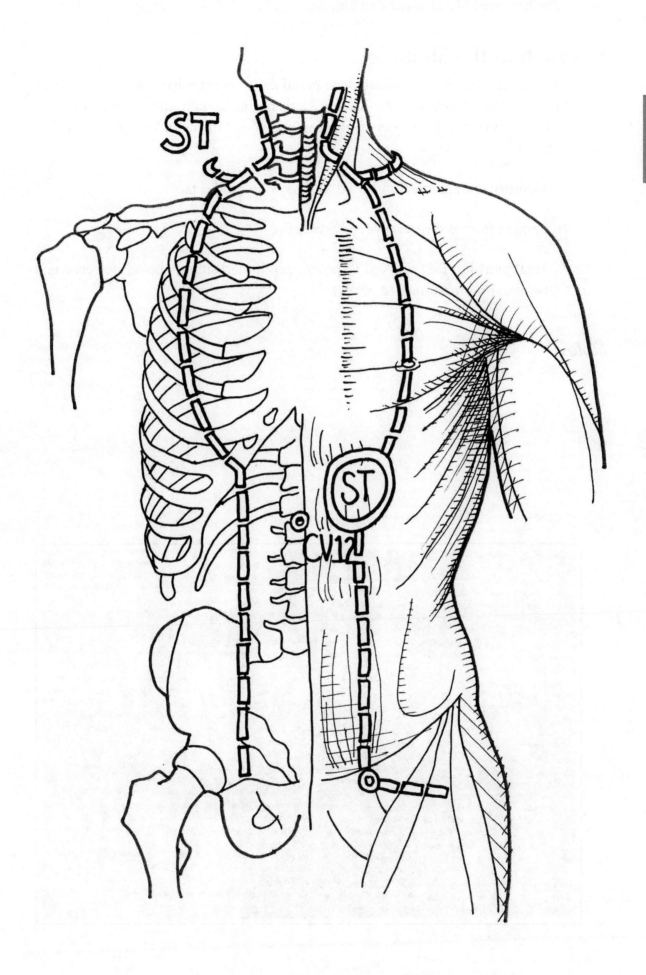

Stomach in the Shoulder

The extended branch of ST which flows round the 'tee-shirt collar' line towards GV14, Big Bone (see Colour Meridian Charts 4), then runs laterally almost horizontally to join the arm via the 'Little Fiery Gate' (two points on Fire meridians) between TH14 and SI10.

Memory tip: Horizontally – like a table: ST = food = table.

This branch is often very reactive and productive.

Treatment tip: Best worked in prone, positioned sitting above the receiver's head to ensure 90-degree access.

Notes

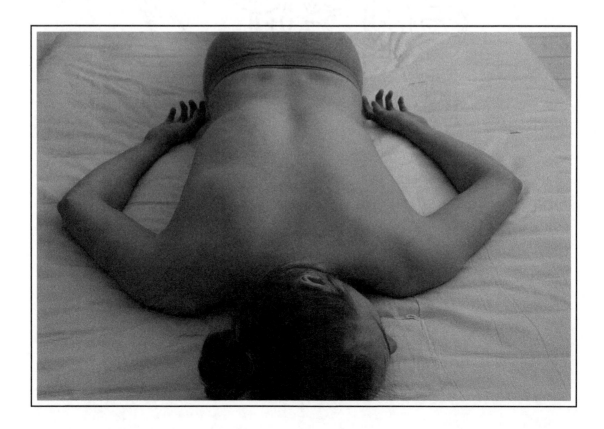

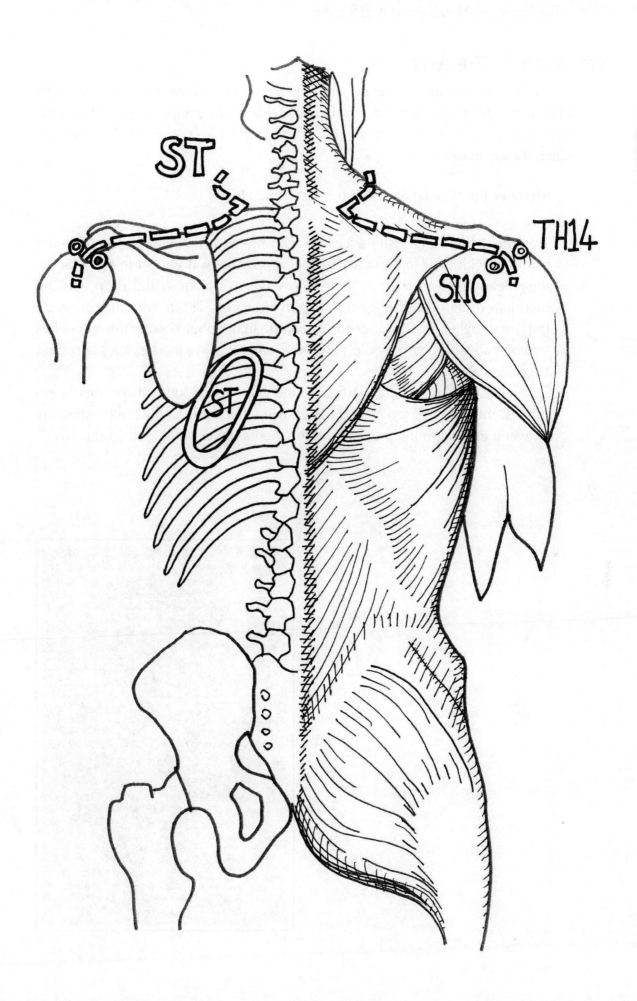

Stomach in the Arm

ST in the arm runs directly parallel and posterior to TH. Below the wrist it takes the line of traditional TH and ends on the ulnar side of the fourth finger. (TH on the Masunaga chart ends on the radial side of the fourth finger – see Colour Meridian Chart 9 for comparison.)

Memory tip: 'The fat Stomach pushes Triple Heater over.'

Treatment tip: ST is easily accessed with the receiver lying supine in 'sling position' with their forearm across their upper hara. If you sit in seiza facing their head you can support their elbow with your knee and drop into the meridian using curved fingertips. (You can access TH in the same position, but use straight fingertips instead of curved.) In the photo below the model has a futon roll where you would have your knee if using the treatment position suggested above.

At the elbow you are skirting round the medial side of the olecranon process (but don't go too medial or you will fall into SI8 in the hollow midway between the olecranon process and the medial epicondyle of the humerus).

Notes

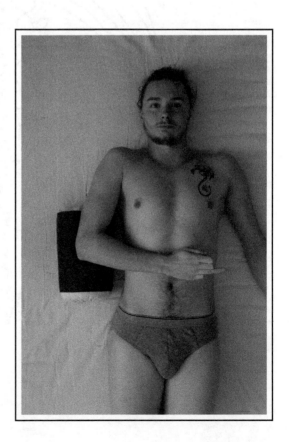

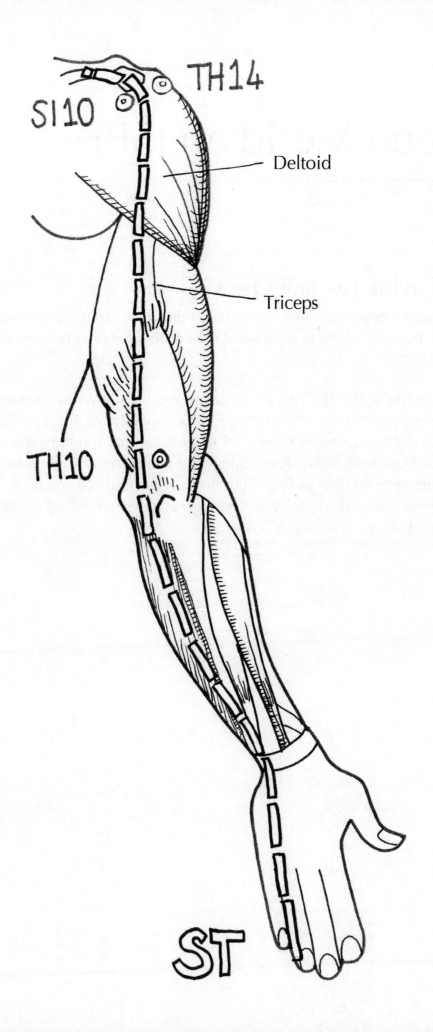

TH14

SI10

Deltoid

Triceps

TH10

ST

Spleen Meridian (SP)

Spleen in the Jaw and Chest

Masunaga's extension of SP takes the line of the lateral portion of traditional ST in the jaw. It then descends the neck just lateral to ST on the anterior part of sternocleidomastoid (SCM).

Treatment tip: The jaw and neck are most easily worked sitting above the receiver with their head cradled in your hand. Rotate the head slightly (about 20 degrees) and for the neck, lift the head so that you bring the meridian up to your thumb rather than sinking your thumb into the meridian: this avoids the uncomfortable feeling of pushing into the throat. If you hook your thumb slightly into SCM you will come accurately into SP rather than working onto ST.

Notes

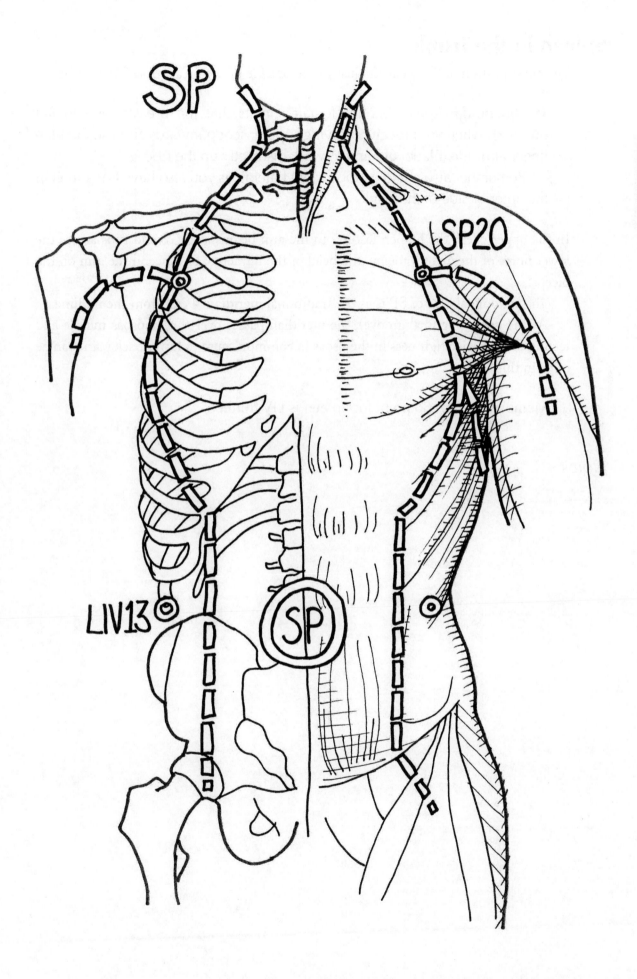

SP

SP20

LIV13

SP

Spleen in the Trunk

The chest portion of SP is curved, just to the outside of the breast tissue in women.

> **Treatment tip:** Remember for female clients that the breasts tend to fall outwards when your receiver is lying supine; scoop inwards and use the little finger and side (blade) of hand to work discreetly up the ribcage.
>
> Remember also not to go too far out (lateral) as you also have LIV and LI in the anterior side of the trunk.

In the upper chest, the branch leading to the arm begins at SP20 and runs across the lower fibres of the deltoid (below the head of the humerus) to descend the arm on the biceps.

The abdominal part of SP is as the traditional meridian: 4 cun from the midline.

At the groin (inguinal groove), the meridian passes over the iliopsoas muscle and testing for excessive tightness in the psoas (a common cause of lower back pain) can be done in this area.

> **Memory tip:** The Bo point for Spleen is LIV thirteen.

Notes

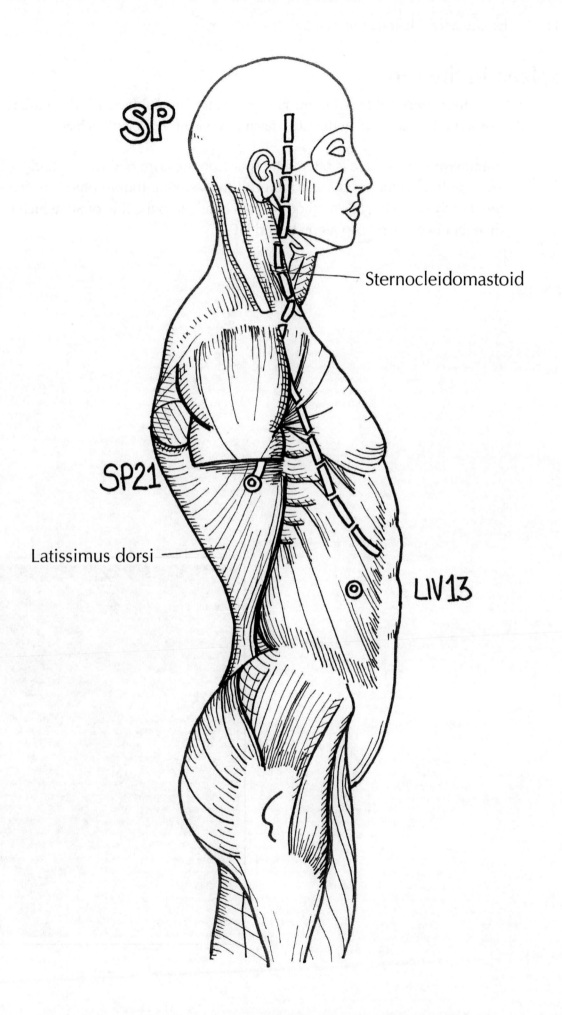

SP

Sternocleidomastoid

SP21

Latissimus dorsi

LIV13

Spleen in the Arm

SP runs directly parallel to LU in the arm but is more medial (towards the midline of the arm). It is best accessed in the LU stretch position at 4 o'clock/8 o'clock.

> **Treatment tip:** As there is often little space on the arm, one way of finding SP accurately is to locate LU and then roll the working thumb onto the side of the thumb tip. Using this method you fall neatly into the line of SP, which can then feel like a 'slot' between LU and HP.

Notes

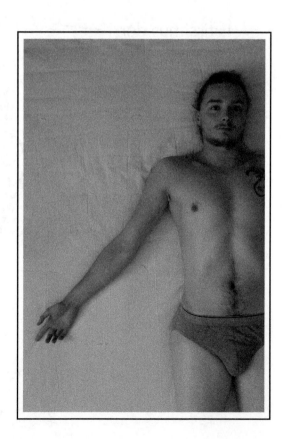

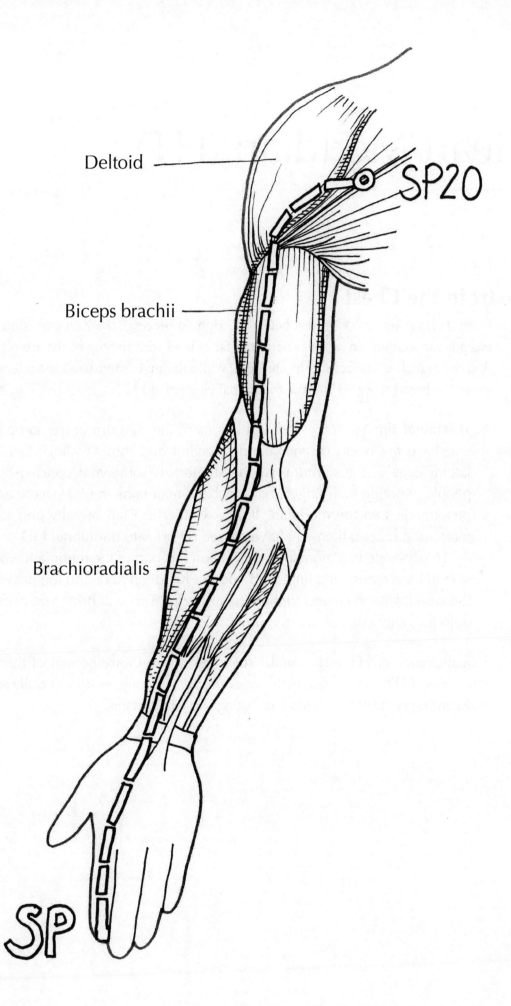

Deltoid

SP20

Biceps brachii

Brachioradialis

SP

Heart Meridian (HT)

Heart in the Chest

From its Bo point at CV14 (just below the xiphoid process), the Zen extension of HT ascends the sternum on its outer border as far as level with the top of the armpit crease. A short branch continues up the sternum, while the main meridian runs laterally just above the breast tissue to join the traditional channel at HT1.

> **Treatment tip:** You can work both sides of the sternum at the same time if you have the backs of your hands together and thus the fingertips on the lateral edge of the sternum. As the sternum is somewhat concave in most people, working with fingers back to back maintains the 90-degree angle of penetration into the meridian. If you wander too far laterally and fall into intercostal spaces, then you have moved off HT into traditional KID.
>
> To penetrate in a more focused way on this part of the meridian, work one side of the sternum at a time with 'mother hand' on hara and the fingertips of the working hand curved slightly towards you. This will bring you accurately onto the outer edge of the sternum.

A small section of HT tucked under the lower jaw and into the root of the tongue reminds us of HT's connection with *communication*. This portion is most easily accessed whilst sitting at the receiver's head and using curved fingertips.

Notes

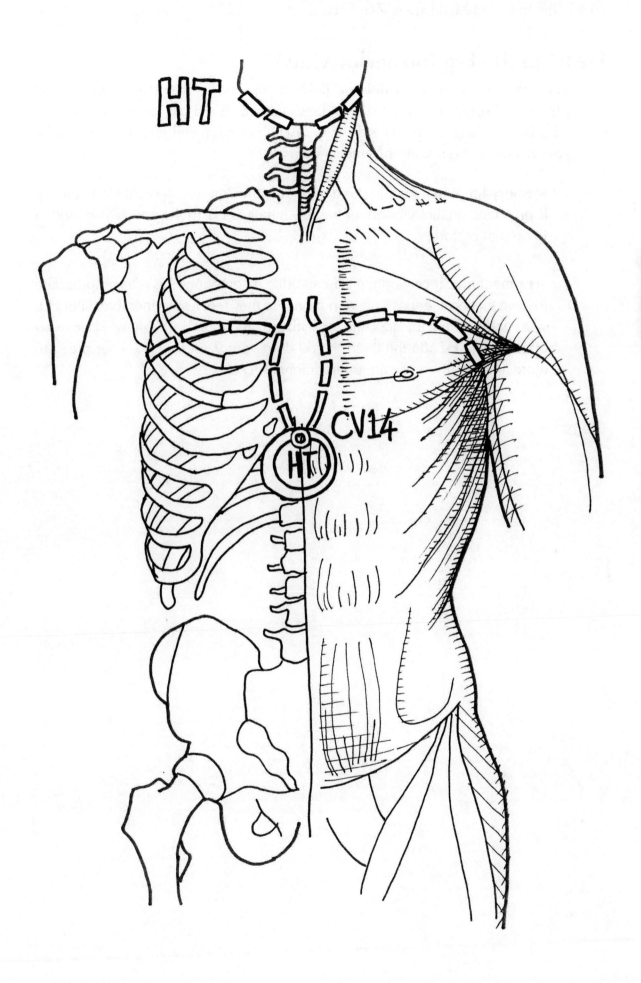

HT

CV14

Heart in the Leg (posterior view)

HT runs very close to traditional KID on the medial hamstrings and medial gastrocnemius, but lies closer to the midline of the thigh and calf (nearer to traditional BL). It runs along the medial side of the Achilles tendon and ends tucked into the centre of the heel (see Colour Meridian Chart 14).

Memory tip: When people stand normally, the Zen extension of HT in the leg is protected on the 'yinside' of the leg, rather as HT in the arm is also hidden in normal posture.

Treatment tip: Since working HT can bring up emotions it is often appropriate to have the receiver positioned in prone, so they feel less vulnerable. Sitting in seiza and working the opposite leg with arm and thumb straight will bring you directly onto HT. (In the thigh, if you drop your wrist to make your pressure more anterior, then you are on traditional KID.)

Notes

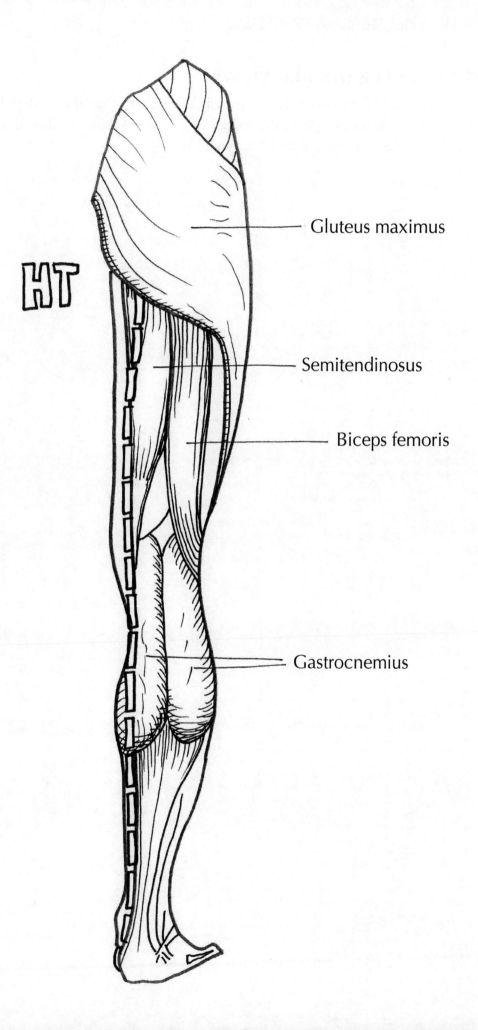

HT

Gluteus maximus

Semitendinosus

Biceps femoris

Gastrocnemius

HT

Heart in the Leg (medial view)

In the lower leg HT runs quite close to the midline of gastrocnemius but slightly on the medial side. It then flows down the medial side of the Achilles tendon, finishing in the centre of the heel (see Colour Meridian Chart 14).

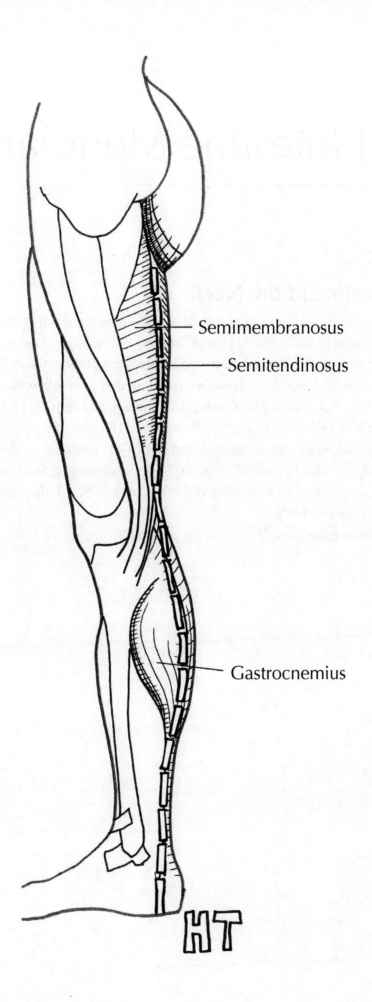

Semimembranosus

Semitendinosus

Gastrocnemius

HT

Small Intestine Meridian (SI)

Small Intestine in the Neck

Several noted Zen Shiatsu teachers speak of SI running along the posterior border of the SCM muscle, and the side view of head on Masunaga's chart certainly shows this. However, we feel the Masunaga map is inconsistent and confusing when we compare the front, side and rear views. Therefore in this drawing we follow the traditional course of SI in the neck running in a straight line diagonally from SI17 round the neck to Big Bone (GV14). If you extend the line from SI18 (under the zygomatic arch directly inferior to the outer end of the eye) and SI17 (just posterior to the angle of the jaw and anterior to SCM), you will cross SCM approximately 1.5–2 cun below the ear. If at this point you find Ki is running down the back of SCM, then follow it till it shifts backwards towards GV14.

A definite occasion to 'feel it out for yourself'.

Notes

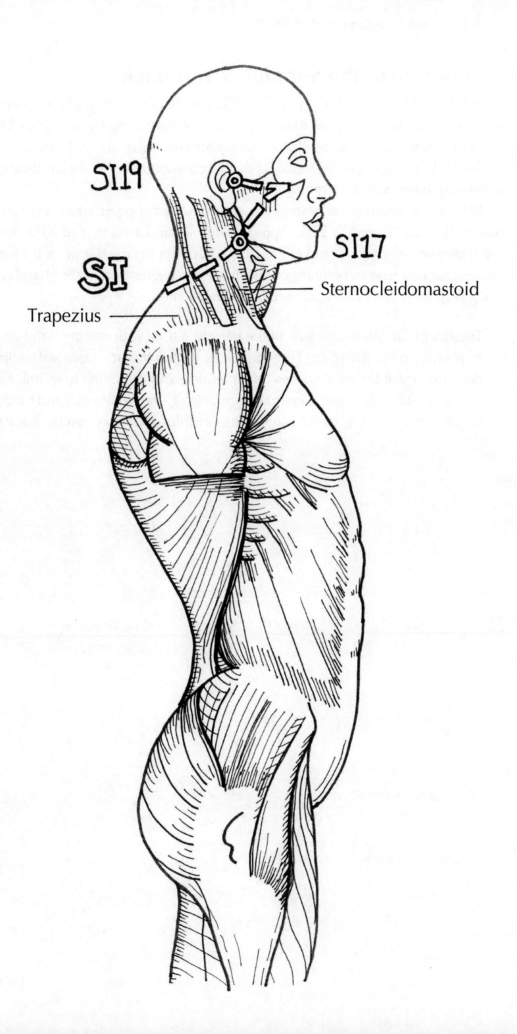

SI19

SI17

SI

Sternocleidomastoid

Trapezius

Small Intestine in the Shoulders and Back

From GV14 ('Big Bone' point, where all the Yang meridians converge), SI runs outwards towards the top of the scapula. Masunaga's map softens the zigzags of the traditional pathway somewhat, but the meridian definitely runs through points SI14 and 13, which we find are important in the treatment of shoulder tension, being on the levator scapulae and supraspinatus muscles respectively.

SI11 in the centre of the scapula is a sensitive 'marker point' which indicates the start of the route down the back. Approximately 2 cun lateral to Zen KID (see text and illustration on pages 66 and 67) SI can be felt from the inferior tip of the scapula, crossing the iliac crest and running on the fullest and highest part of the gluteal region, going deep about level with the lower end of the sacrum.

Treatment tip: Work one side of the back at a time with mother hand on SI11 to tune in to the meridian. Fingertip work on the thoracic area will help you drop into the intercostal spaces (often tender) and switching to thumb for the buttocks will assist you in penetrating through gluteus maximus and medius to the piriformis muscle, which is often responsible for referred lumbar back pain.

Notes

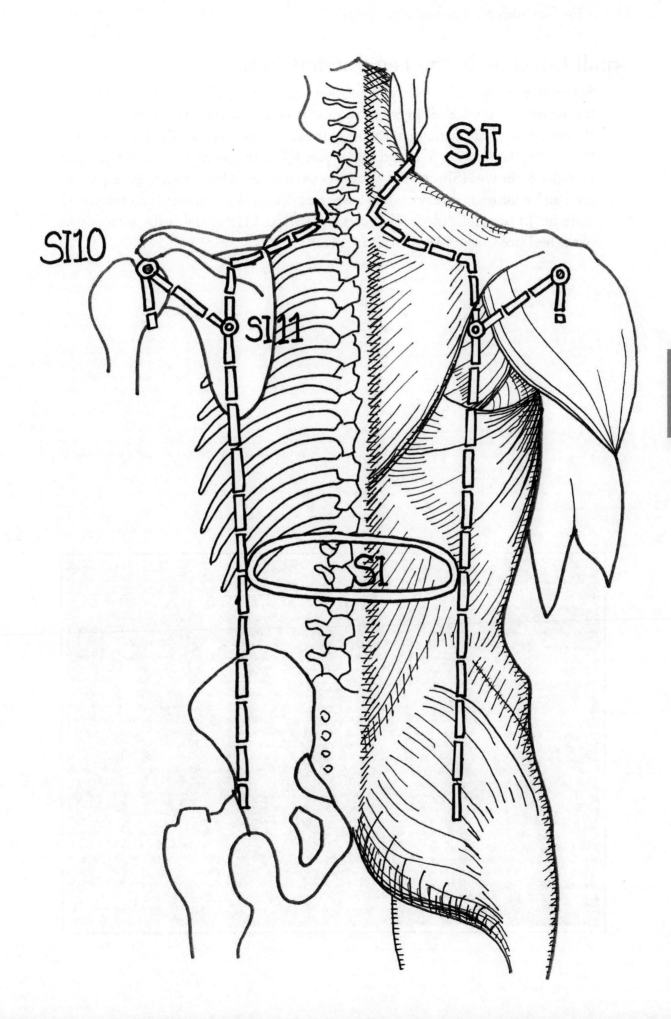

Small Intestine in the Leg (medial view)

SI is most easily worked in its stretch position 'heel to knee', which will help distinguish it from SP 'toe to ankle'. SI in the thigh runs along the medial edge of quadriceps. At the knee it runs just anterior to the most prominent part of the epicondyle of the femur (LIV8 being just *posterior* to it) and then proceeds into the groove between the palpable posterior of the tibia (SP) and the gastrocnemius muscle. SI here often feels deep to the giver and sensitive to receiver in the lower part. Running just posterior to the medial maleolus, SI curves slightly forward, crossing KID and HP to end at the anterior part of the heel (see Colour Meridian Chart 14).

Notes

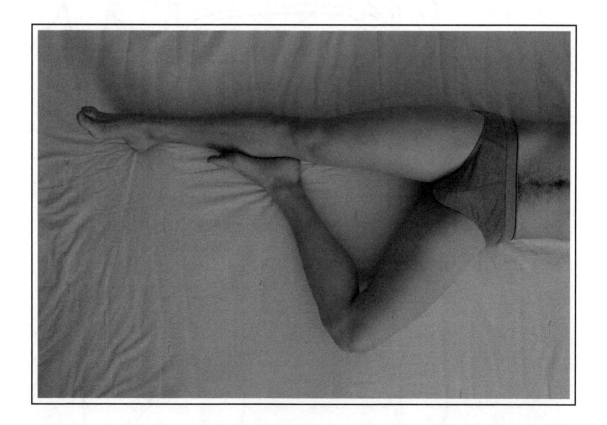

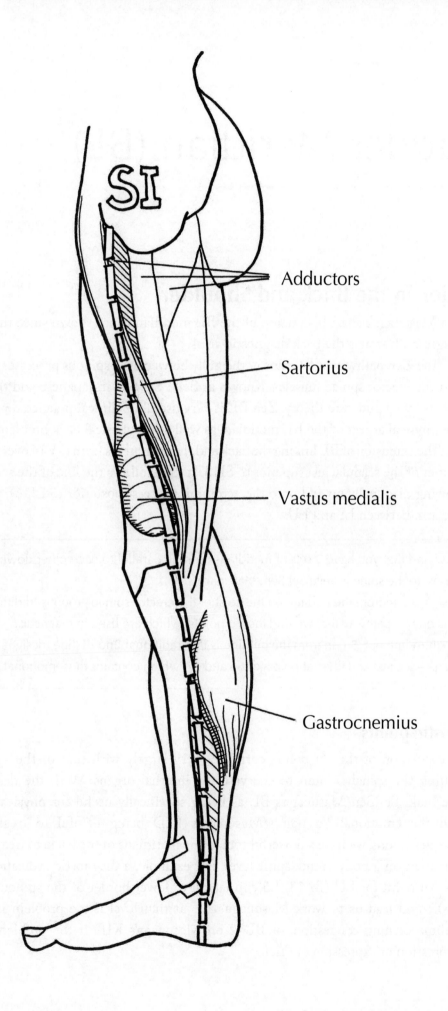

SI

Adductors

Sartorius

Vastus medialis

Gastrocnemius

Bladder Meridian (BL)

Bladder in the Back and Shoulder

On Masunaga's chart his version of the BL meridian is not shown since the back view diagram illustrates the back diagnostic areas.

The Zen pathway of BL runs in the gully between the spinous processes of the spine and the erector spinae muscles. Known as Seiki Sei Sen in Japanese and the Hua Tuo points in acupuncture theory, Zen BL is very useful in clinical practice for working on the physical aspect of the BL meridian, as well as on physical back problems.

The extension of BL linking the back and the arm curves from GV14 over the superior corner of the scapula, just superior to SI13. It then follows the line of the scapular spine flowing diagonally up and onto the acromion process (posterior to LI16), to drop into the arm between LI and LU.

> You now find that you have 3 sets of meridians running parallel to each other down the back.
>
> Closest to the spine is Seiki Sei Sen: Masunaga's BL.
>
> Next, 1.5 cun from the midline on the crest of the erector spinae group is traditional 1st BL line. It is on this pathway that we find the Yu points, which are used in diagnosis.
>
> The third line out, 3 cun from the midline is the traditional 2nd BL line (designated KID by Masunaga – see text and illustration pages 66 and 67) which contains the 'emotional Yu points'.

Diagnostic points

The position of the Yu points correlates very largely with that of the spinal nerves exiting the spinal column to enervate the internal organs. With the designation of the Seiki Sei Sen/Masunaga's BL as being specifically useful for physical imbalance and the emotional Yu points/Masunaga's KID being helpful to treat emotional manifestations, we have a powerful tool in the meridians of the back, to treat any organ/meridian on a body–mind–spirit level. For example, a diagnostic indication found at the Yu point for LU (BL13, 1.5 cun lateral to lower border of the spinous process of T3) could lead us to work Masunaga's BL at that level if the problem involved say, asthma or lung congestion, or BL42 on Masunaga's KID if the problem was more depression or expression of grief.

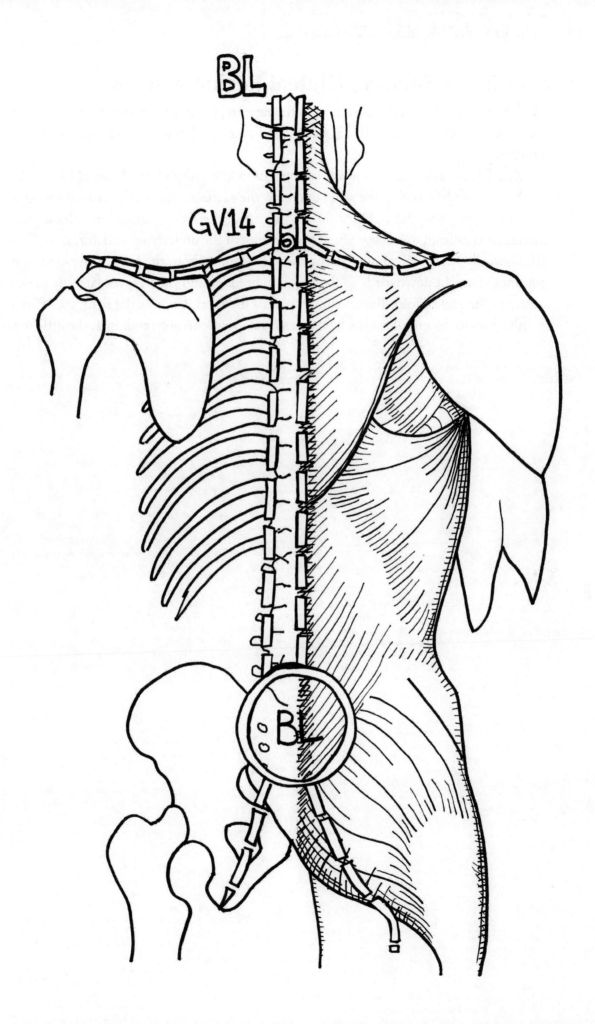

BL

GV14

BL

Bladder in the Sacrum, Gluteal Region and Leg

Traditionally the BL meridian runs onto the sacrum just slightly medial to the posterior superior iliac spine (SI and BL Yu points are found here) then zigzags onto the sacral foramina.

Zen BL is rather more simple, coming from the gully close to the spine in the lumbar area and following the same line onto the sacrum. Often, due to excess weight in the area, or particular tightness in the origins of the erector spinae muscles on the sacrum, it is difficult to be clear about the location of the underlying structures, but Zen BL is usually fairly easily found in the sacral foramina. From the base of the sacrum it continues straight downwards to the ischial tuberosity and then moves laterally to the centre of the gluteal fold. The remaining part of the meridian is as the main traditional pathway down the middle of the hamstrings and gastrocnemius, ending at the little toe.

Notes

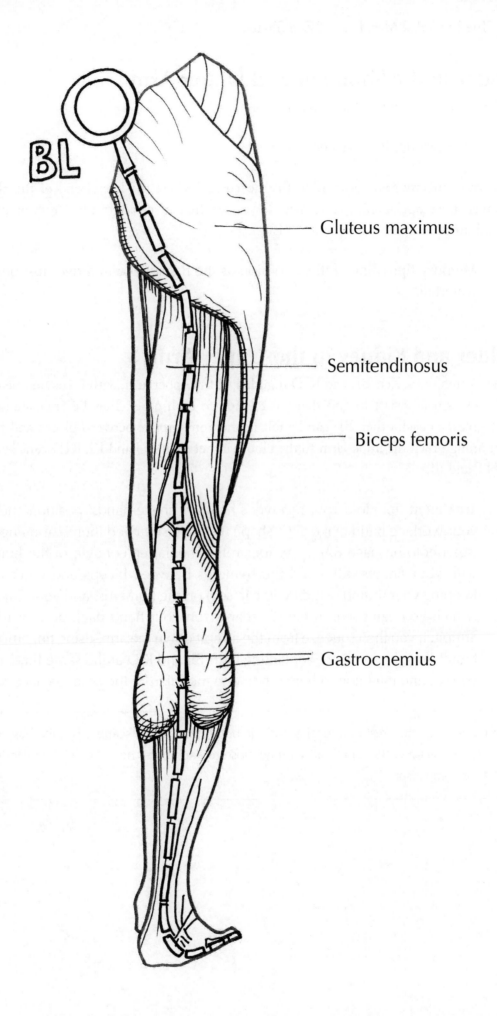

BL

Gluteus maximus

Semitendinosus

Biceps femoris

Gastrocnemius

BL

Bladder in the Shoulder and Upper Arm

BL follows the line of the scapular spine.

Memory tip: BL = Water = bones.

It runs directly *posterior* to LI16 (in the 'corner' where the lateral end of the clavicle meets the scapular spine), and then flows over the flat surface of the acromion process and drops onto the arm *anterior* to LI15.

Memory tip: Think of the acromion as the flat surface in a river just before a waterfall.

Bladder and Kidney in the Upper Arm

We often work Zen BL and KID together in the upper arm, with focus on one or the other, as it is easiest to find them in relation to each other. They lie opposite (at 180 degrees) to each other. BL can be felt in the bony groove between biceps and triceps running down the upper arm to the elbow, in between LU and LI. KID runs between HT and SI.

Treatment tip: Hold your receiver's hand in 'shake hands' position and with your working hand make a 'C' shape using outstretched thumb and fingertips (see photo on page 62). Now locate the medial epicondyle of the humerus with your fingers (KID) and the humerus between biceps and triceps (BL). Keeping your thumb (which you can see) on the humerus, and your fingertips (which you can't see) in the 'C' shape, run your hand back up towards the armpit. If you then squeeze from the armpit down the arm, using fingertips and thumb together, you are contacting both BL and KID at the same time. Focus your Ki and intention to home in to one meridian or the other as necessary.

> The area between the crest of trapezius and the bony spine of the scapula is quite busy with (from the top) TH, ST, BL, and SI all running close to each other here. See Colour Meridian Chart 4 for comparison.

Notes

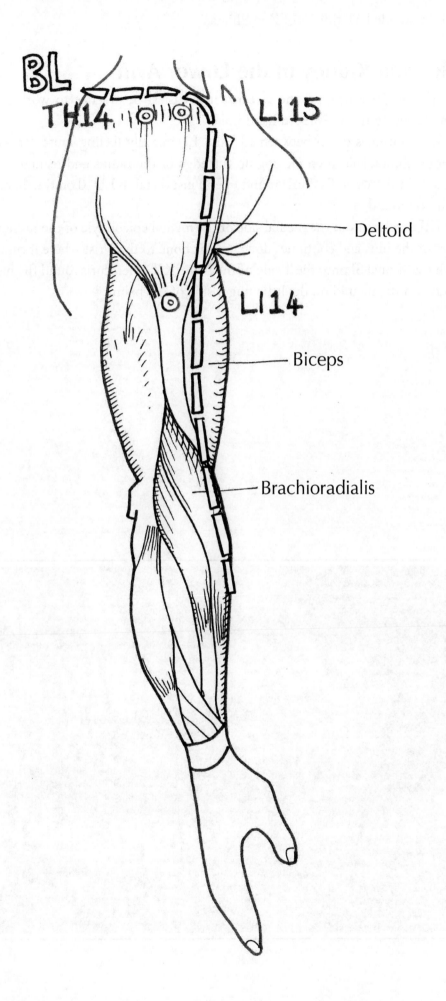

BL

TH14

LI15

Deltoid

LI14

Biceps

Brachioradialis

Bladder and Kidney in the Lower Arm

As in the upper arm, for the forearm it is easiest in practice to work BL and KID together using the 'C'-shaped hand hold.

BL continues down between LU and LI, initially feeling muscular where it runs over brachioradialis, then picking up the edge of the radius and feeling bony down to the side of the wrist. BL curls round to end just distal to LU10 on the thenar eminence (thumb mound).

KID crosses from the medial side of the medial epicondyle of the humerus onto the edge of the ulna and continues down on the bone to the wrist where it runs concurrent with traditional SI onto the 'blade' of the hand. KID then curls round the pisiform bone to end on the mound on the little finger side of the palm.

Notes

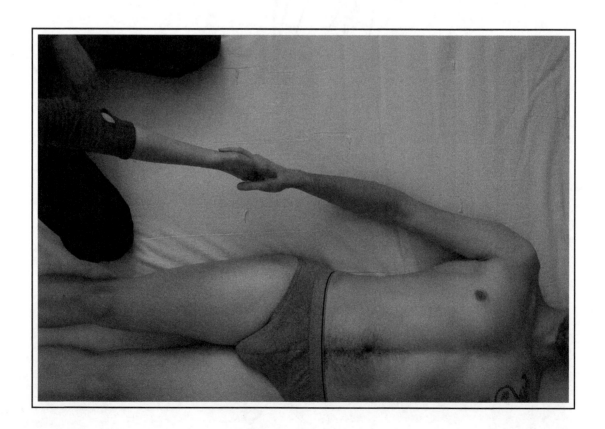

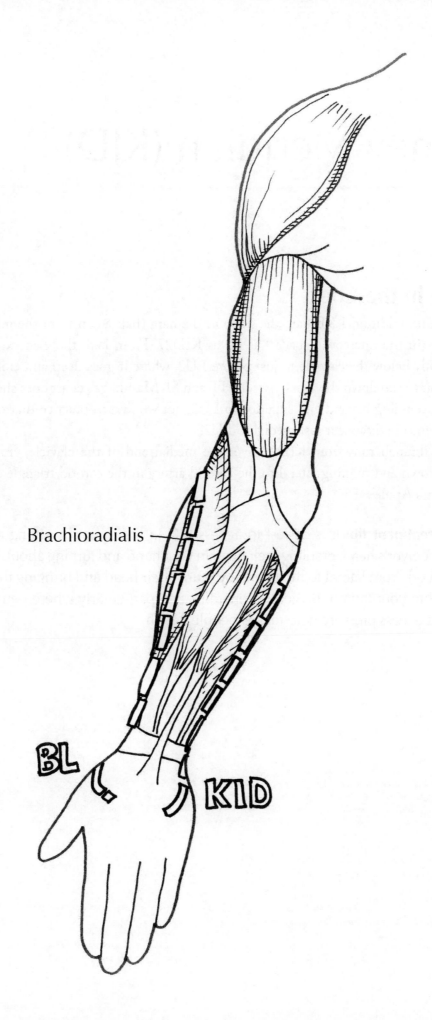

Brachioradialis

BL

KID

Kidney Meridian (KID)

Kidney in the Chest

Zen and traditional KID are the same in the hara (half a cun from the mid line) and chest (in the intercostal spaces) as far as KID27. From here the Zen extension runs laterally below the clavicle to just before LU2, where it goes deep and emerges in the armpit to run down the arm between HT and SI. Masunaga's chart does show the KID line extending beyond and superior to LU2, but we find in practice that often the Ki feel tends to disappear just medial to LU2.

A branch runs from KID27 over the medial end of the clavicle, crossing SCM low down and running lateral to the carotid artery in the carotid triangle as far as the 'Adam's Apple'.

> **Treatment tip:** It is easiest to access KID in the throat by sitting above your receiver's head, cradling their head in your hand and turning about 10 degrees. Work from lateral to the larynx by lifting their head and bringing the meridian onto your thumb. Be gentle generally, and particularly where you cross SCM as excess pressure here makes people cough.

Notes

64

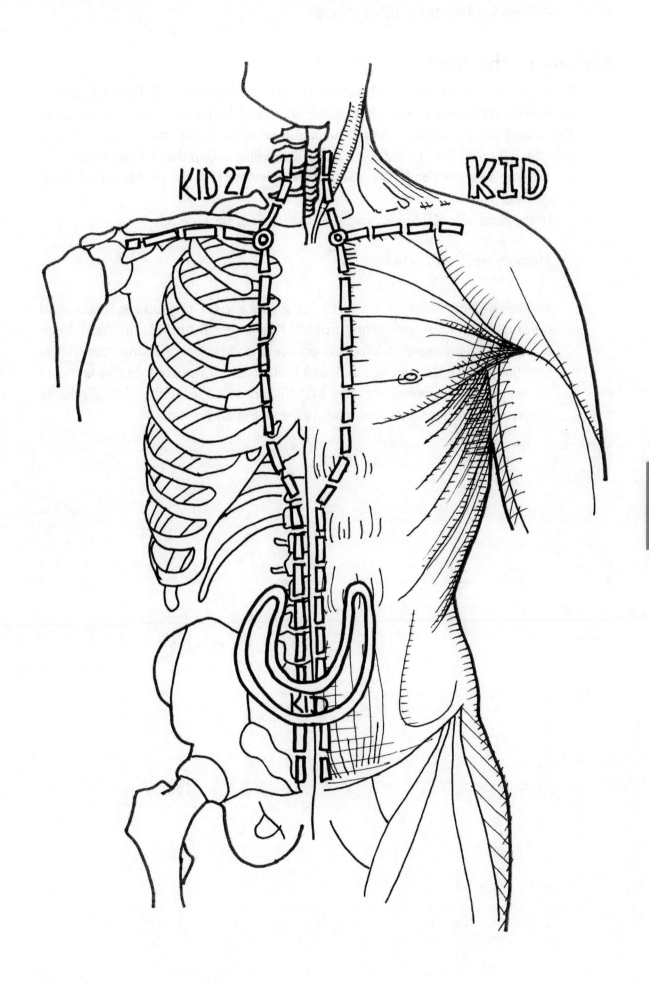

KID 27

KID

KID

Kidney in the Back

Masunaga designated the second traditional BL in the back to the KID meridian. This fits in with traditional thought in that the 'emotional Yu points' lie on this meridian. Emotions being deeper and a more Yin manifestation tie in with the Yin of the Water pair, the KID meridian. Found 3 cun from the midline and in the intercostal spaces in the thoracic area, the Zen KID meridian is felt just lateral to the erector spinae group of muscles.

In the sacral area KID runs along the outer edge of the sacrum.

Memory tip: Water = bones.

Treatment tip: For receivers with lower back pain the lumbar and sacral portions of KID are particularly fruitful. Ki is often disturbed and 'held' here, resulting in tight muscles. Working deeply but sensitively tucking your thumb into the edge of the sacrum (it almost feels like at 45 degrees but in fact is at 90 degrees to the bone) accesses KID Ki and can release the gluteal muscle origins which sometimes feel fearful of relaxing and resting.

Notes

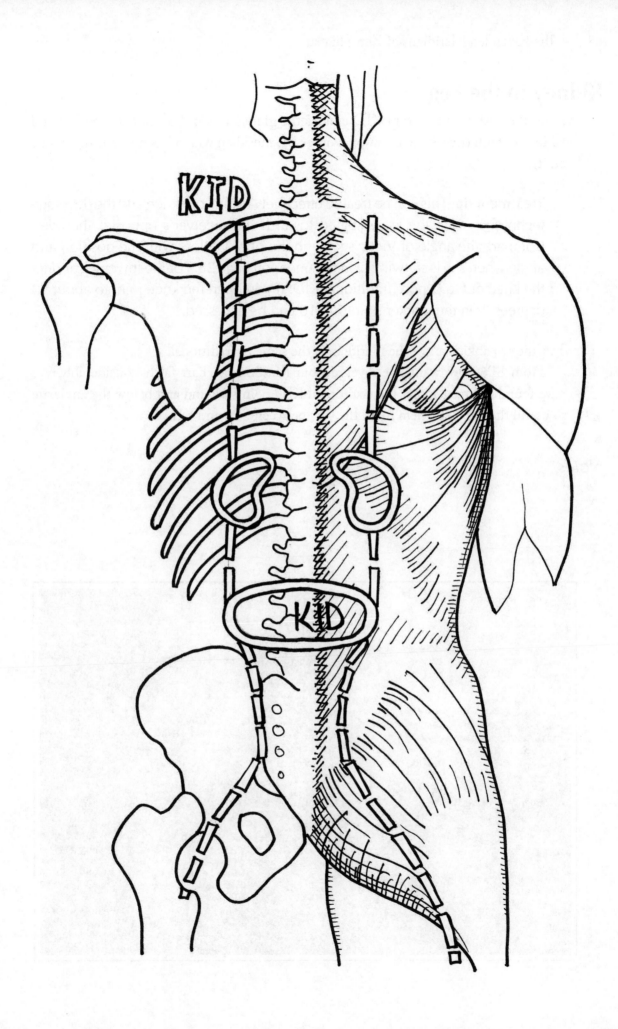

Kidney in the Leg

From the base of the sacrum KID crosses the gluteal mound to run between LU and LI in the thigh (this is the traditional outer BL meridian which has no needling points on it).

> **Treatment tip:** This can be treated effectively using your knee and the 'leverage technique', with the knee angled towards the receiver's opposite shoulder. Compare the angle of Vicky's knee in the photo below with the position and angle when she is showing LI in the photo on page 26. For the lower leg abduct the knee out to expose traditional KID: if you open the knee joint to about 90 degrees then the marker point KID10 can be accessed.

The knee to ankle part of the meridian is the same as traditional.

From SP6 downwards we diverge from Masunaga's chart fairly considerably. We have found in practice that the traditional KID points around and below the ankle are so useful that we take them in on the way between SP6 and KID1.

Notes

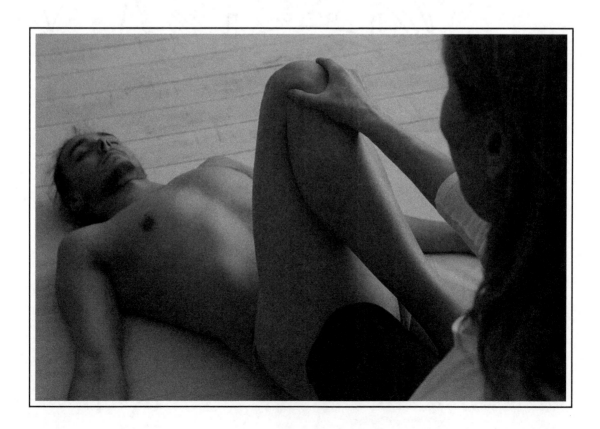

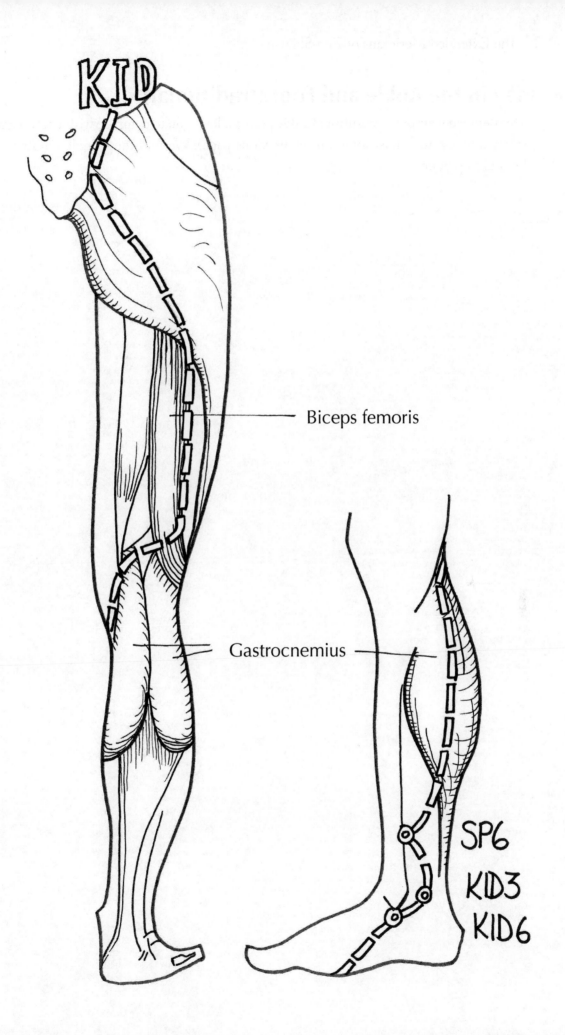

KID

Biceps femoris

Gastrocnemius

SP6

KID3

KID6

Kidney in the Ankle and Foot (traditional)

This detailed view of the traditional ankle points allows you to compare with Masunaga's softer flowing line (illustration on the previous page). We find these ankle points very helpful in practice.

Notes

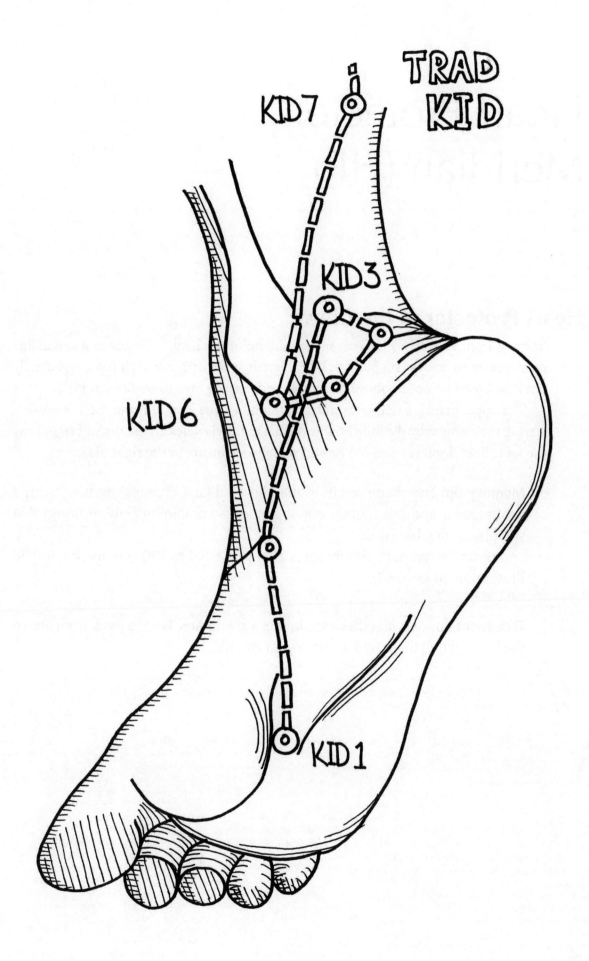

TRAD
KID

KID7

KID3

KID6

KID1

KID

Heart Protector Meridian (HP)

Heart Protector in the Chest

Starting from its diagnostic area on the midline of the hara, HP runs in a single line up the chest to its own Bo point, CV17. Here it splits with a branch running laterally onto the breast tissue just above the nipple and curving over to traditional HP1.

The upper branch swells out on the sternum to cross Zen HT and then re-crosses, leaving the sternum by the little hollow medial to the clavicles. In the throat HP follows the same line; if you can feel the carotid pulse here you are in the right place.

Memory tip: The shape of HP in the chest is like a champagne flute, with a central stem and tall slightly curving sides – containing bubbly liquid that stimulates sociable Fire!

HP on the sternum and throat is always medial to KID (compare with the illustration on page 65).

Treatment tip: As with other anterior neck meridians, best to work from above the head, lifting the meridian onto your thumb.

Notes

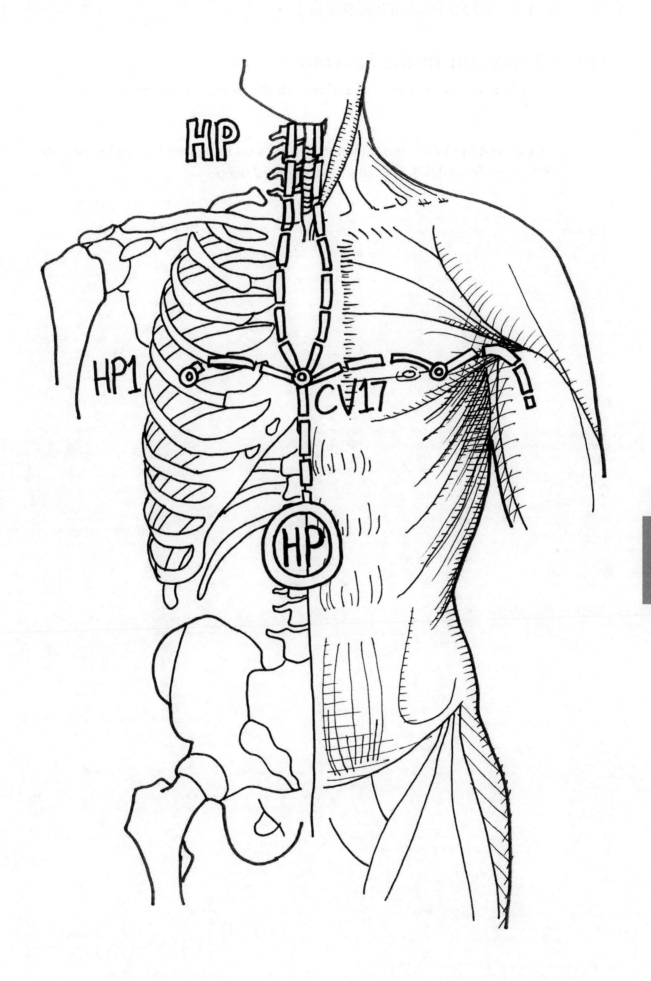

HP

HP1

CV17

HP

HP

Heart Protector in the Sacrum

A short but very useful branch of HP runs in the gluteal area lateral and parallel to Zen KID.

> **Treatment tip:** While the KID meridian runs on bone (see text and illustration on pages 66 and 67), HP feels muscular and deep.

Notes

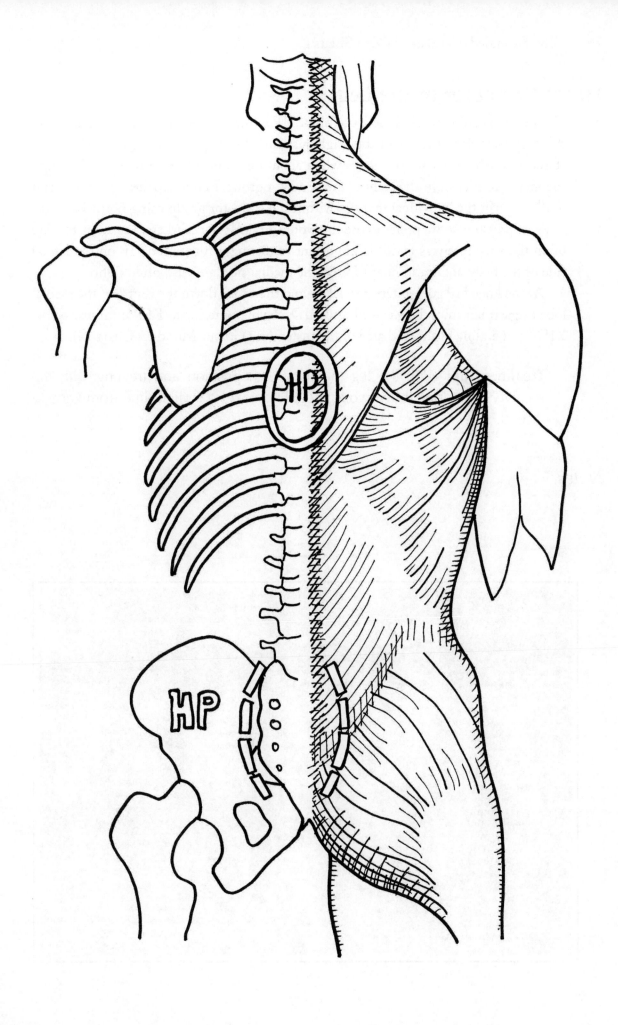

HP

Heart Protector in the Leg

The stretch position we find most useful for HP is 'instep to knee'. This allows access to the deep triangle at the top of the thigh, just lateral to the adductor group, where HP starts, and helps keep at 90 degrees when about one third of the way down the thigh the meridian runs onto the belly of the adductor group. In our experience it is difficult to distinguish the individual muscles within the adductor group using normal Shiatsu levels of pressure, so we prefer to use the whole group as our markers. The adductors are often tight for receivers and it is important to distinguish between HP on the lateral side of the belly, and traditional LIV, on the medial side, and also often tight.

At the knee HP goes anterior to LIV8 and then runs down the centre of the medial lobe of gastrocnemius, between SI and KID, staying anterior to KID until just below KID3 and ending in the mid area of the instep (see Colour Meridian Chart 14).

> **Treatment tip:** With the leg in this stretch position and treating with the receiver's leg draped over your knee, HP makes a straight line from knee to its end.

Notes

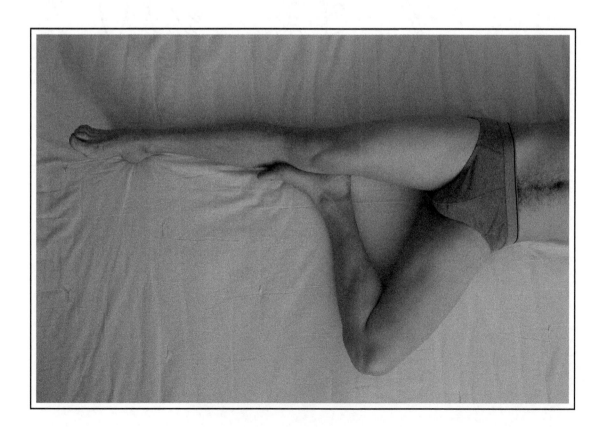

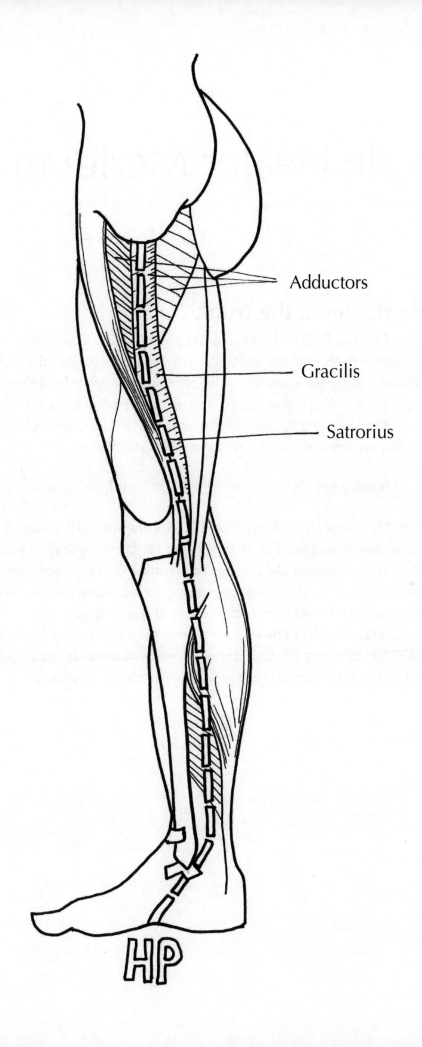

Adductors

Gracilis

Satrorius

HP

Triple Heater Meridian (TH)

Triple Heater in the Trunk

Zen TH runs from its traditional end point (TH23) at the eyebrow, to in front of the ear and deviates from the traditional pathway in that it omits the useful part close round the back of the ear. However, its branch under the ear, behind the mastoid process and up onto the skull following the line of the temporal bone, has a close physical and functional link to the lymphatic system in that we can often feel enlarged lymph nodes in this area when receivers have ear and throat infections.

Memory tip: TH is associated with the lymphatic system in Zen Shiatsu theory.

The Masunaga chart shows Zen TH crossing over GB relatively higher up on the neck than traditional TH. It runs down the posterior scalene muscle on the side of the neck (which feels like a stringy band behind GB) and continues along its traditional pathway just posterior to the crest of trapezius heading for the marker point TH14 in the posterior dimple of deltoid when the arm is abducted.

In the trunk TH flows downwards on 'the back of the side' (if we imagine the body as a 'cornflakes box') as far as the waist, where it comes forwards over the anterior iliac crest. This is the mirror image of LI (see illustration on page 25).

Notes

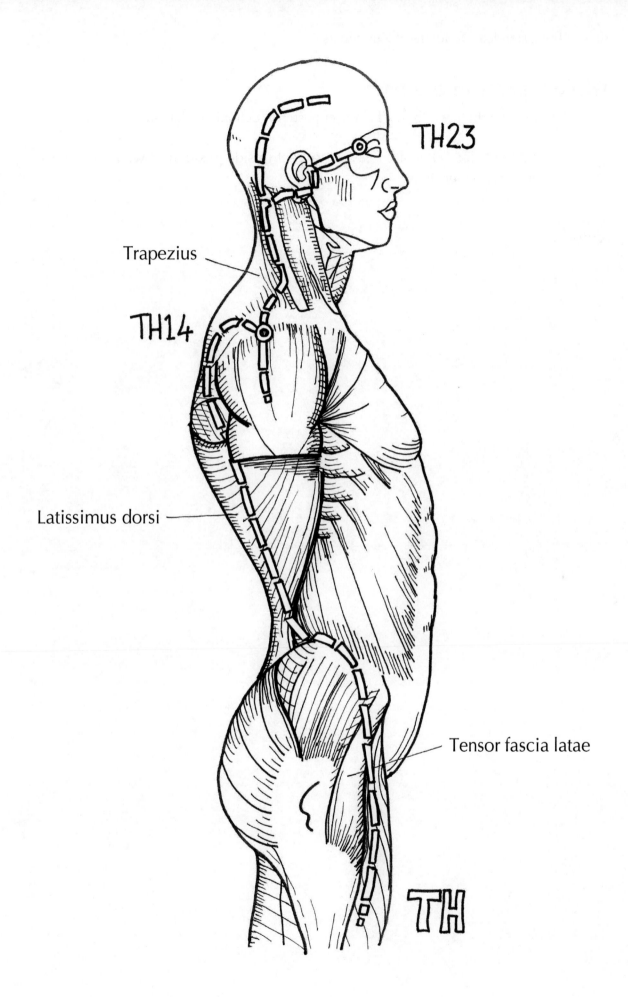

TH23

Trapezius

TH14

Latissimus dorsi

Tensor fascia latae

TH

TH

Triple Heater in the back

TH runs straight down from TH14 over posterior deltoid and latissimus dorsi.

Treatment tip: TH is often easiest to treat in side position as we have access to the entire meridian.

Notes

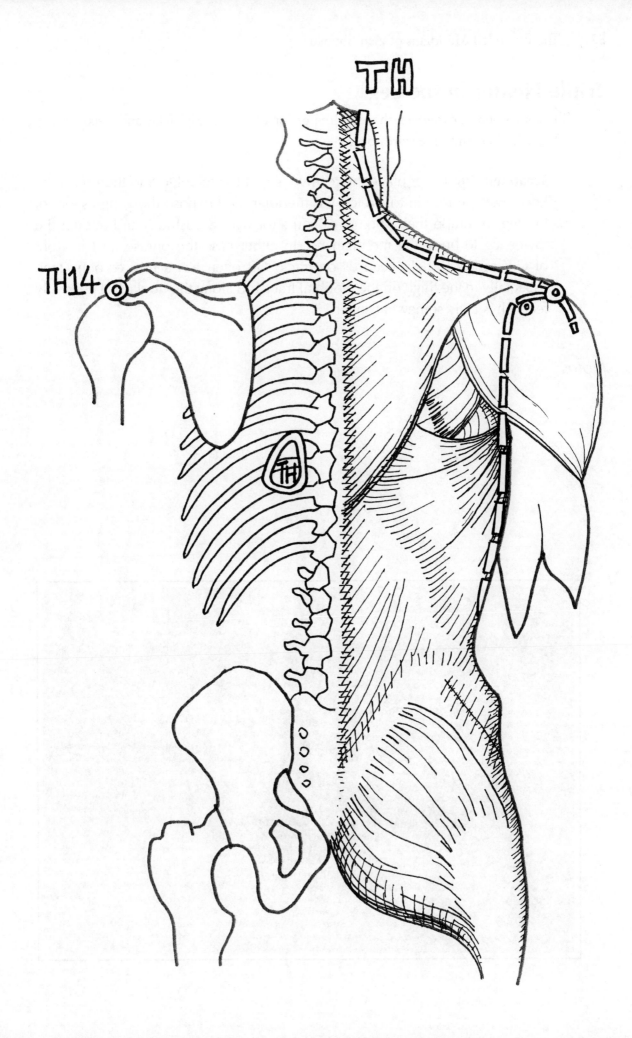

TH

TH14

TH

Triple Heater in the Leg

TH comes onto the thigh on the anterior portion of tensor fascia latae and runs between ST and GB down to the third toe.

> **Treatment tip:** Either place the receiver's foot toe to ankle and then push the knee away from you to stretch the meridian and expose the yang aspect of the leg, or drape their knee over yours (or over a cushion) and abduct the lower leg to bring the meridian up. In either case the phrase 'just in front of GB' seems to help keep us on track. GB often has a firm or bony feel, especially in the thigh on the iliotibial tract and along the fibula: TH generally feels physically somewhat softer.

Notes

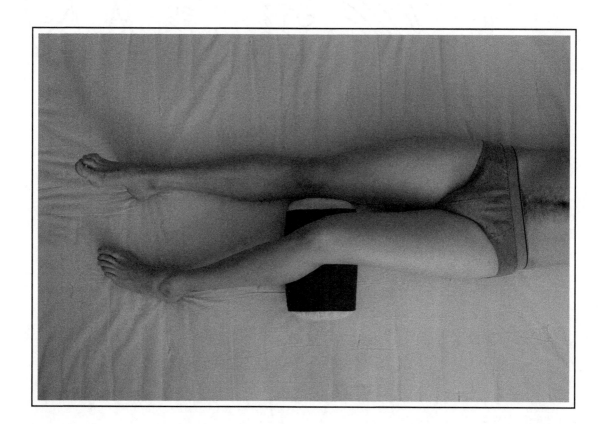

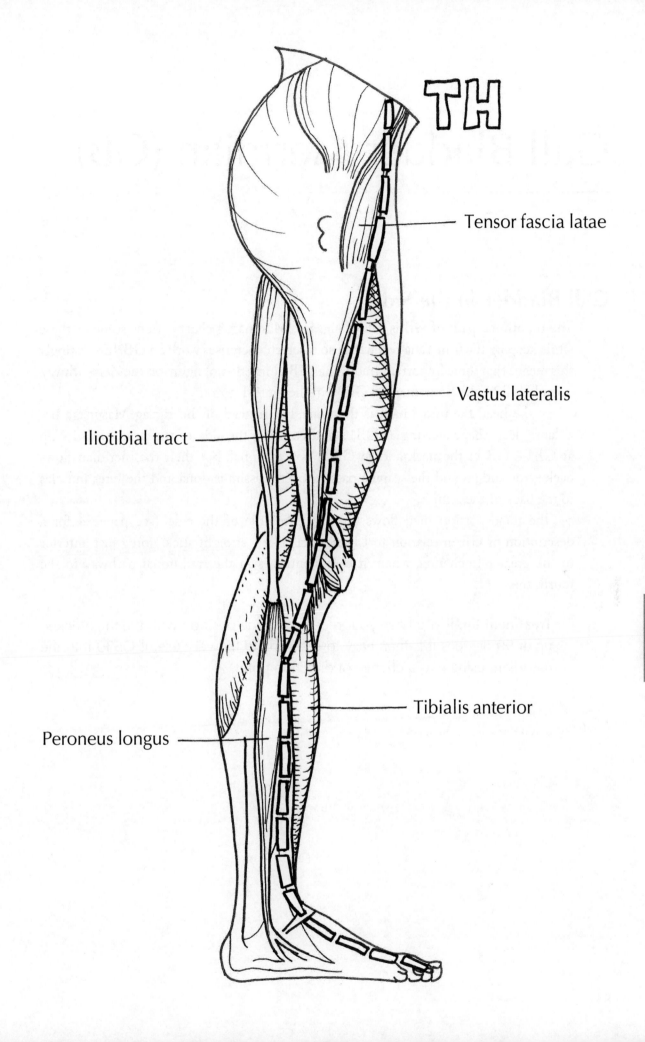

TH

Tensor fascia latae

Vastus lateralis

Iliotibial tract

Tibialis anterior

Peroneus longus

Gall Bladder Meridian (GB)

Gall Bladder in the Side

The traditional path of GB is full of zigzags. Masunaga's chart softens some of these while keeping the firm Yang feel which so often characterises work on GB. Interestingly this means that some important traditional GB points do not figure on the Zen pathway, notably GB24, the Bo point, and GB30 in the gluteal region.

In the head the initial path is the same, but instead of the zigzag Masunaga has a 'laurel leaf' shape starting at GB19 and covering the side of the head, with its tip at GB14. GB in the neck and to GB21 is traditional, but then the meridian flows backwards and around the scapula passing over latissimus dorsi and the teres muscles to the back of the armpit.

The torso portion then flows down 'the middle of the side' (see page 24 for a description of GB in relation to LI and TH) like a straight stick, going just anterior to the greater trochanter, where it then continues in the traditional pathway to the fourth toe.

Treatment tip: If you have your receiver in side position with the thigh flexed up at 90 degrees it is then easy to incorporate the very useful GB30 into the meridian, using it as a change of direction point.

Notes

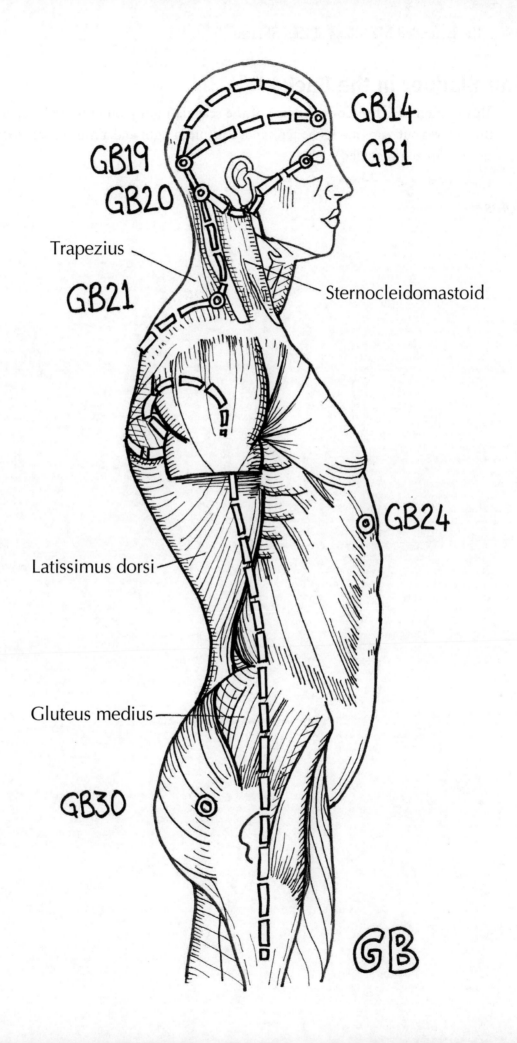

GB14
GB1
GB19
GB20
Trapezius
Sternocleidomastoid
GB21
GB24
Latissimus dorsi
Gluteus medius
GB30
GB

Gall Bladder in the Back

This portion of GB follows the line of the scapula right around to its lateral edge. It then moves outwards along the teres muscles (often tight and a fruitful area to work in cases of 'frozen shoulder').

Notes

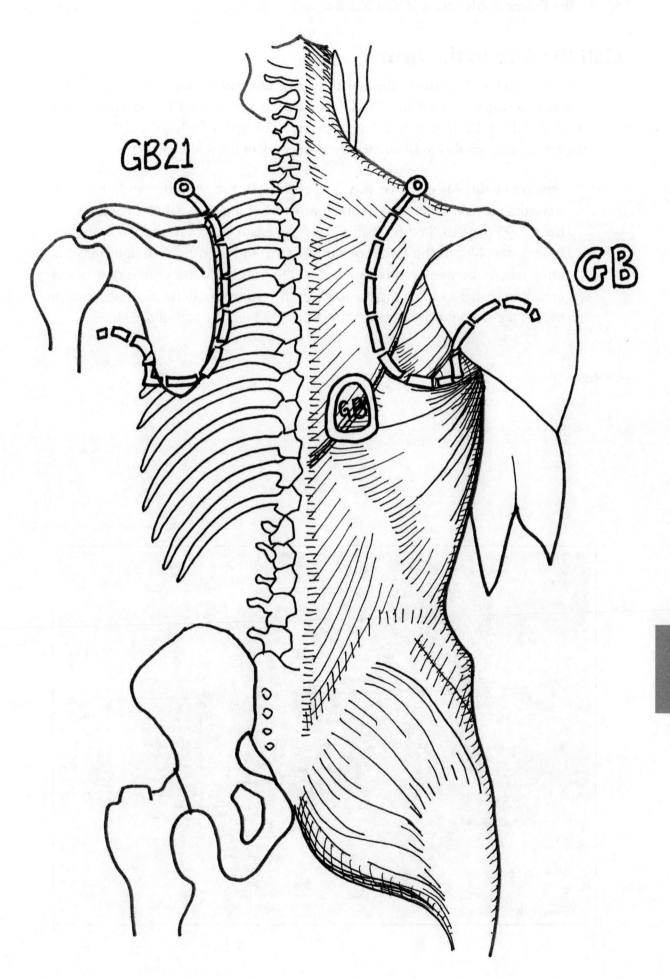

GB21

GB

Gall Bladder in the Arm

From the back of the armpit, the branch of Zen GB which flows into the arm goes through the 'Big Fiery Gate' (SI10 and SI9) and crosses SI, ST and TH on the posterior portion of deltoid. It then turns before it reaches LI14 (apex of deltoid) and flows down the arm directly parallel to LI all the way to the back of the middle finger.

> **Treatment tip:** An effective way to treat GB in the shoulder and arm is to have the receiver lie prone with their arms reaching above their head, elbows bent at 90 degrees. In this position you can easily work around the scapulae, thumb deeply into the posterior armpit area and then flow straight into the arms where the meridian is exposed in the middle of the visible part of the arm. Remember to angle slightly towards the radius to catch GB in the forearm (not in the deep groove between the bones, which is traditional TH).

Notes

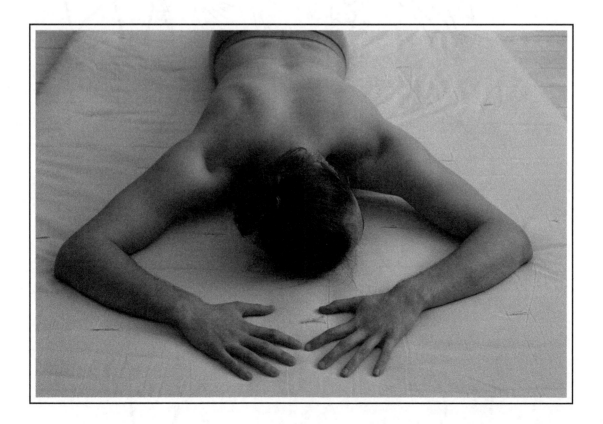

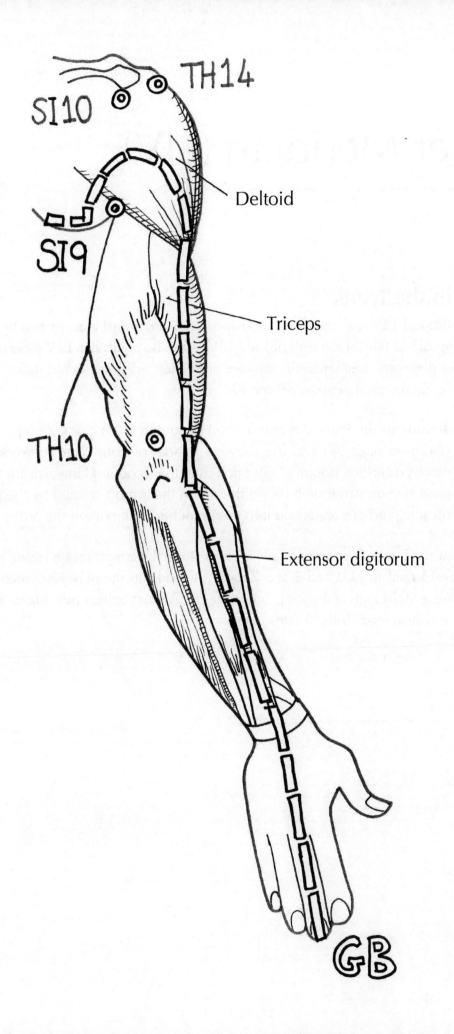

SI10

TH14

Deltoid

SI9

Triceps

TH10

Extensor digitorum

GB

Liver Meridian (LIV)

Liver in the Trunk

Traditional LIV makes a diamond shape in the abdominal area, its two upper points being LIV13 (end of eleventh rib) and LIV14, the Bo point. Zen LIV picks up the flow at its diagnostic area (and mirror image on the left side), misses out its Bo point, and curves up the chest between SP and LI.

> **Treatment tip:** Place the arm in the LIV stretch (10 o'clock/2 o'clock: see the photo on page 94) and use the side 'blade' of your hand to work LIV in a more posterior 'chopping' direction than the 'scooping' inwards for SP. In this position you can thumb round the rim of the armpit created by the pectoralis muscle, and this leads you into the branch running down the arm.

From the front of the armpit, LIV ascends along the armpit crease (think of a raglan sleeve) lateral to LU1 and 2 and Zen SP. It heads up the neck just anterior to GB, crossing SCM high and ending below the ear. A short branch runs horizontally from the meridian towards the Adam's Apple.

Notes

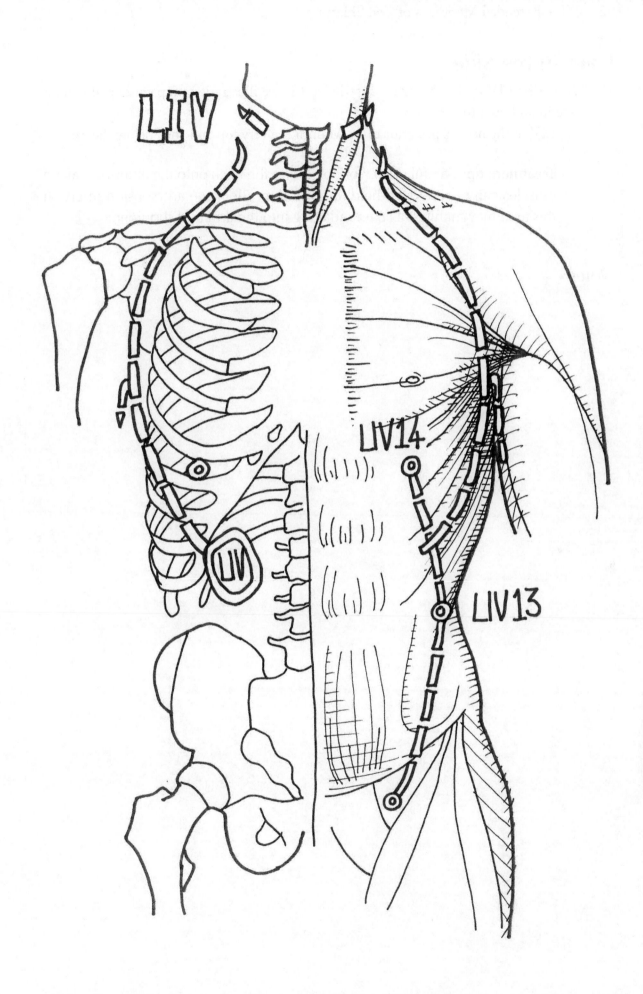

LIV

LIV14

LIV13

LIV

Liver in the Side

Note that LIV in the chest runs anterior to LI (see illustration on page 25 and Colour Meridian Chart 6).

LIV in the neck is posterior to SCM until the very top and ends below the ear.

Treatment tip: Careful deep work on LIV in the neck onto the anterior scalene muscles can release deep-held neck tension. Blockage and tension in LIV in this area may manifest as pain radiating into the arm and shoulder.

Notes

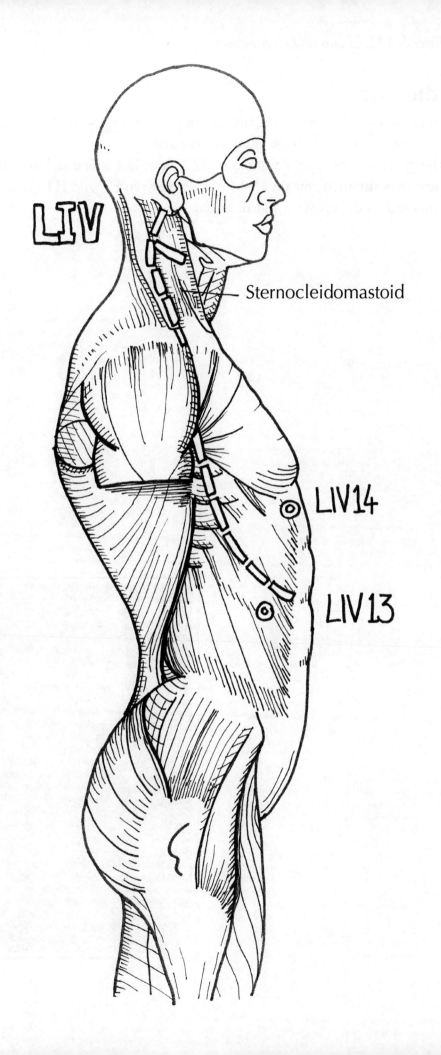

LIV

Sternocleidomastoid

LIV14

LIV13

Liver in the Arm

The Zen extension is best treated in the stretch position (10 o'clock/2 o'clock), which allows continuity of work from the chest into the arm.

In the upper arm the meridian runs in the groove just lateral to biceps (with the arm in stretch position). Below the elbow it flows between HP and HT on the forearm flexors, and ends at the tip of the fourth finger.

Notes

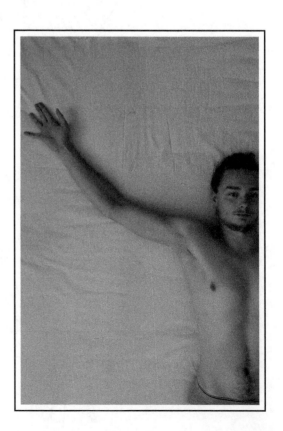

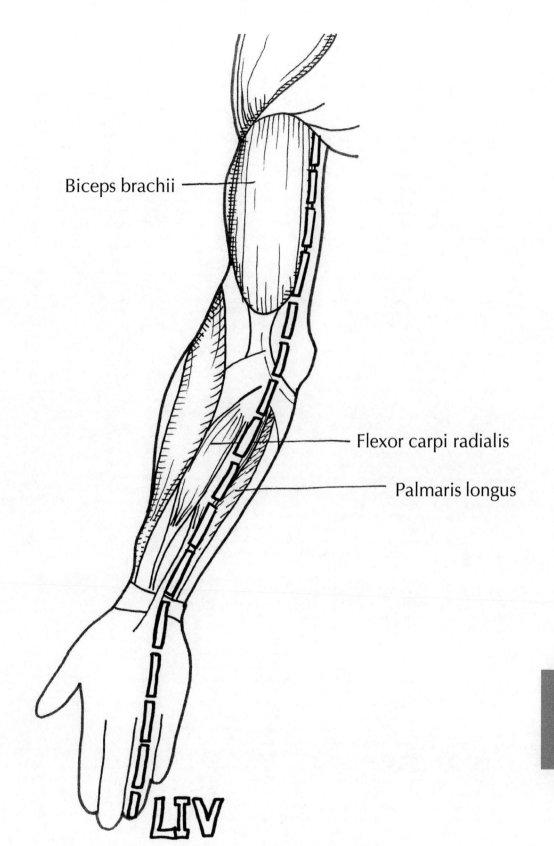

Biceps brachii

Flexor carpi radialis

Palmaris longus

LIV

Colour Meridian Charts

1. Back Diagnosis Chart

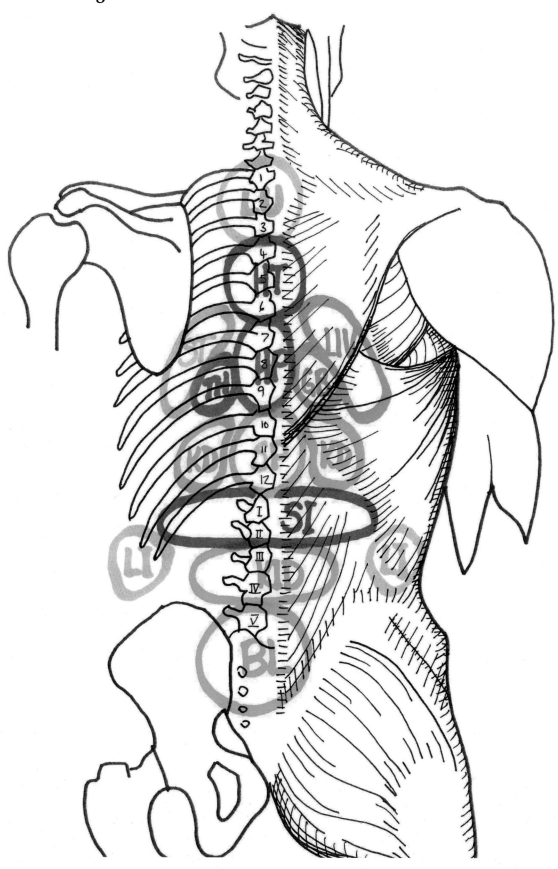

2. Hara Diagnosis Chart

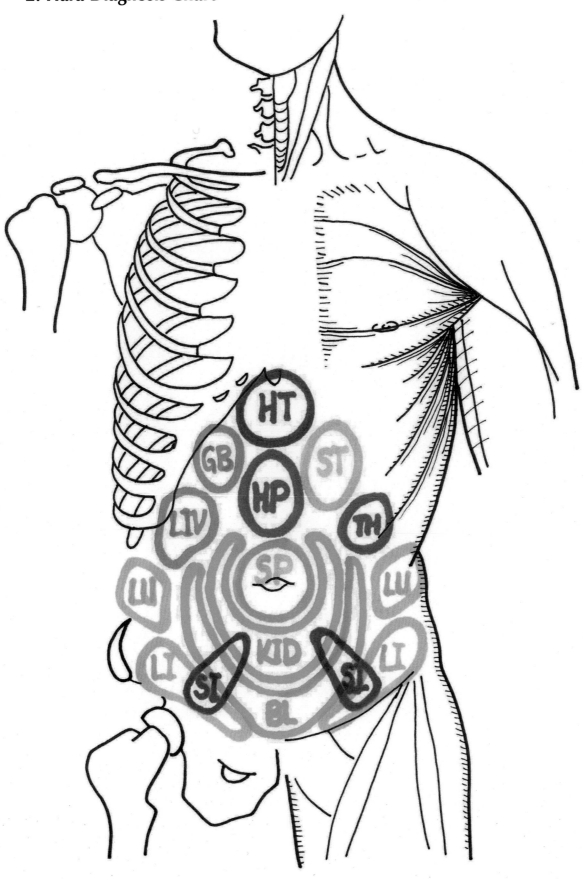

3. Hara Diagnosis Areas and All Anterior Trunk Meridians

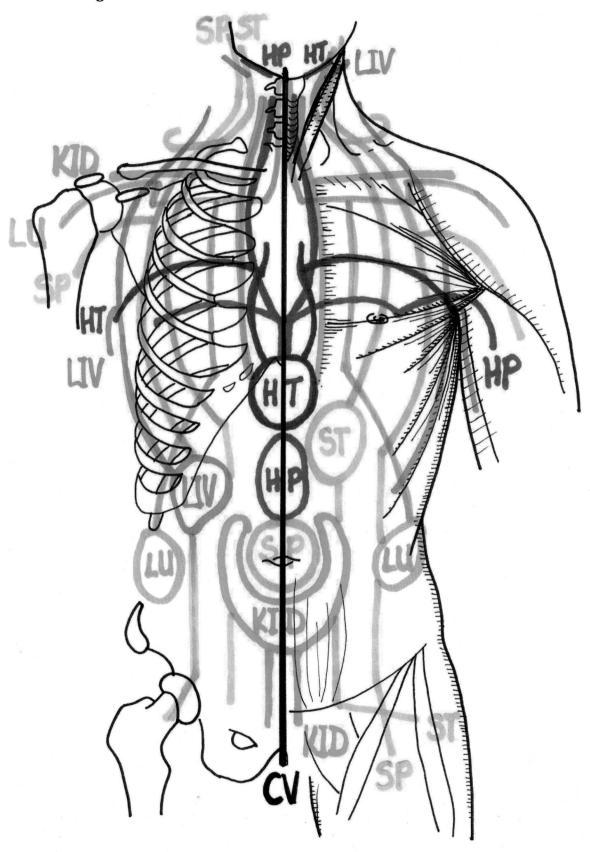

4. Back Diagnosis Areas and All Posterior Trunk Meridians

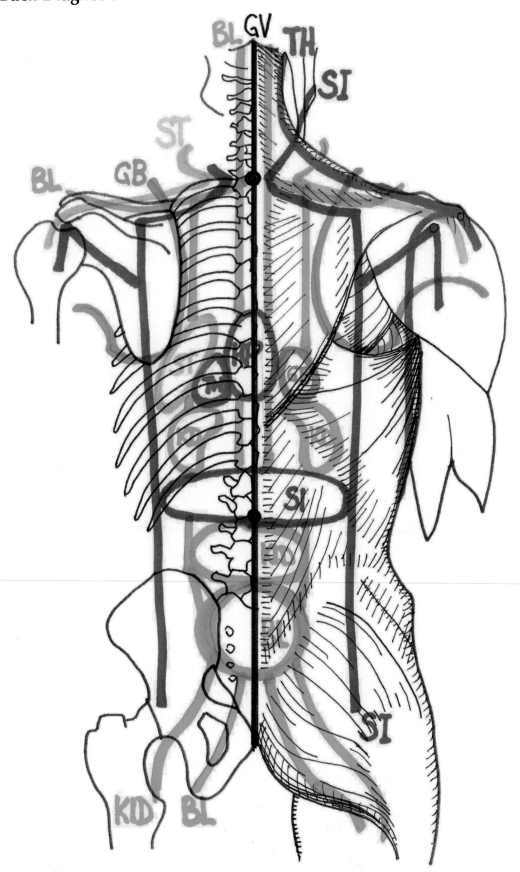

5. Side of Head and Neck Meridians

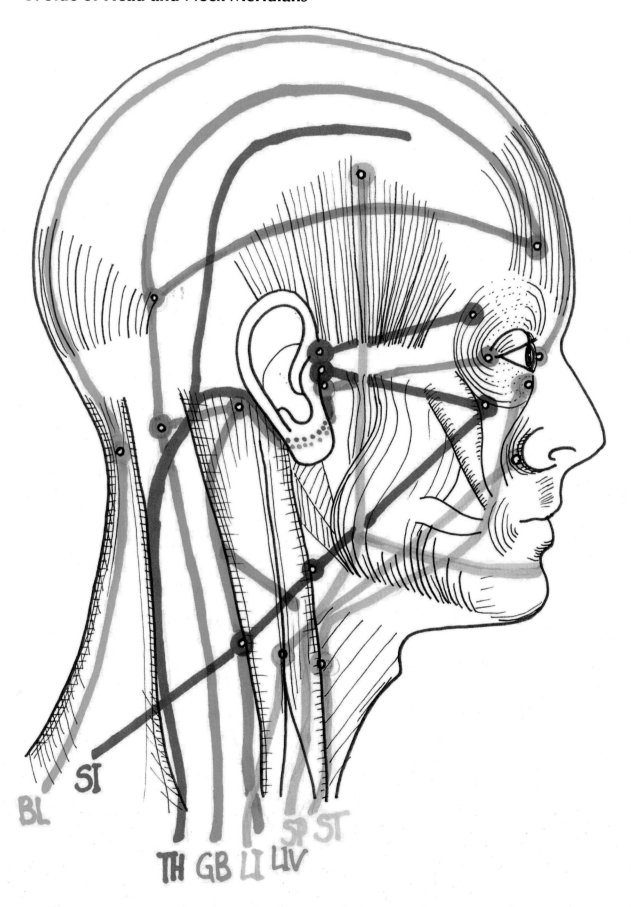

SI

BL

TH GB LI LIV

SP ST

6. Side of Body All Meridians

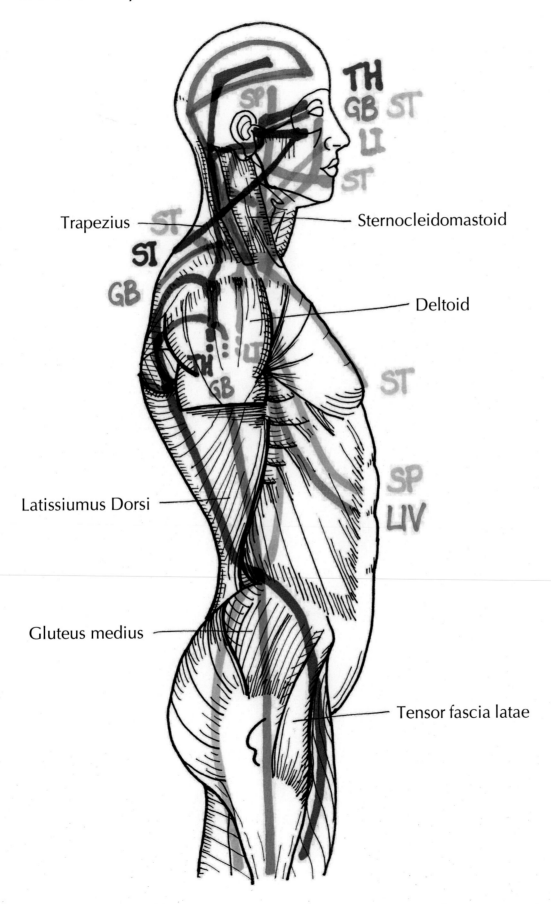

TH
GB ST
LI
ST

Trapezius — ST ————— Sternocleidomastoid

SI

GB

Deltoid

TH LI
GB

ST

Latissiumus Dorsi —

SP
LIV

Gluteus medius —

Tensor fascia latae

7. Anterior Arm All Meridians

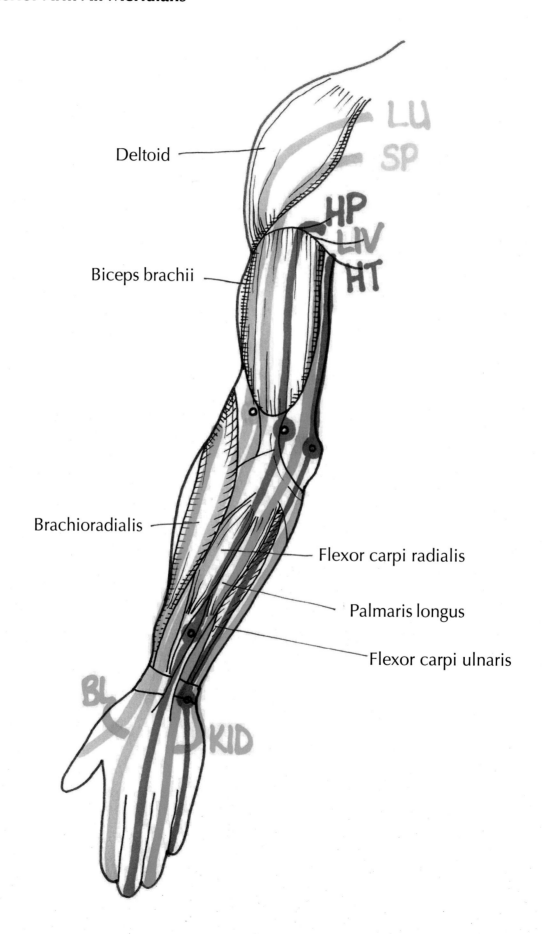

Deltoid

LU

SP

HP

LIV

HT

Biceps brachii

Brachioradialis

Flexor carpi radialis

Palmaris longus

Flexor carpi ulnaris

BL

KID

8. Lateral Arm All Meridians

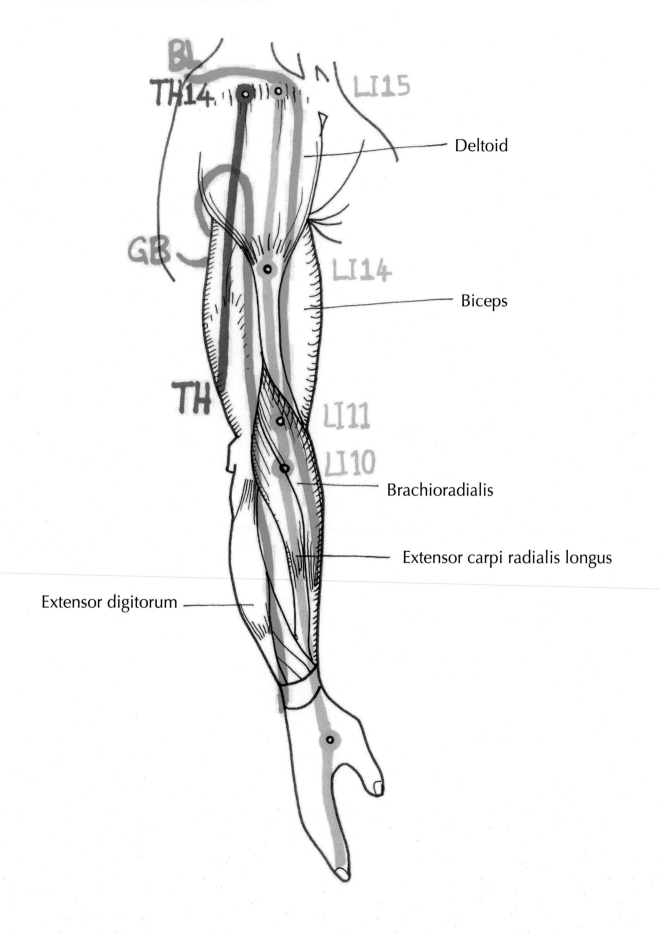

BL

TH14

LI15

Deltoid

GB

LI14

Biceps

TH

LI11

LI10

Brachioradialis

Extensor carpi radialis longus

Extensor digitorum

9. Posterior Arm All Meridians

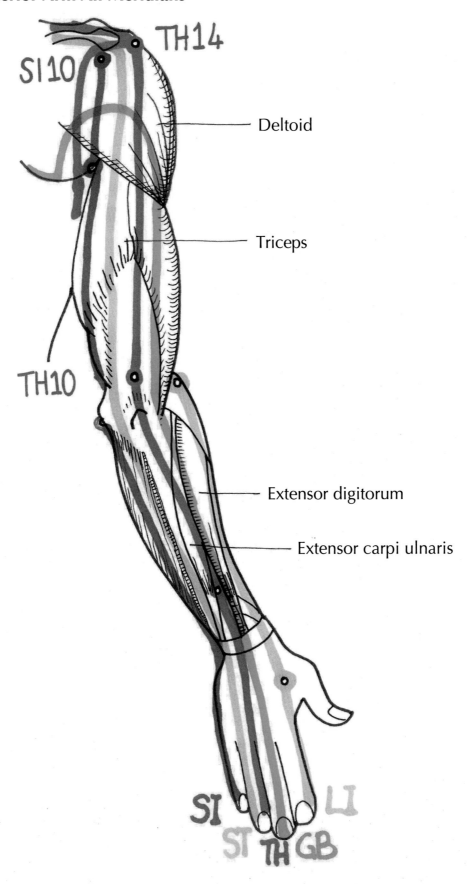

TH14

SI10

Deltoid

Triceps

TH10

Extensor digitorum

Extensor carpi ulnaris

SI

LI

ST

TH GB

10. Anterior Leg All Meridians

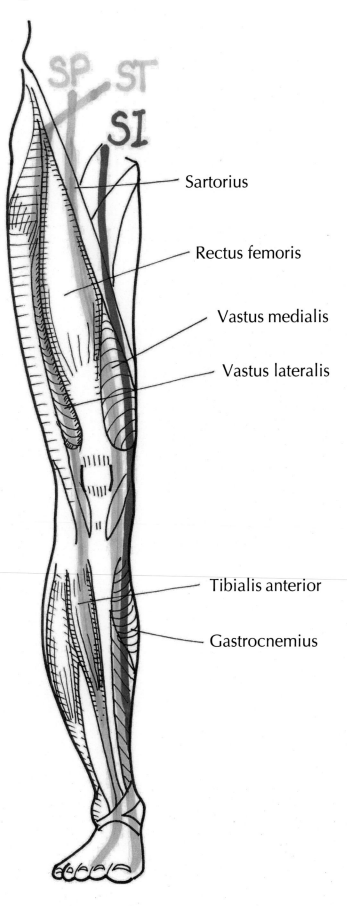

SP ST

SI

Sartorius

Rectus femoris

Vastus medialis

Vastus lateralis

Tibialis anterior

Gastrocnemius

11. Lateral Side Leg All Meridians

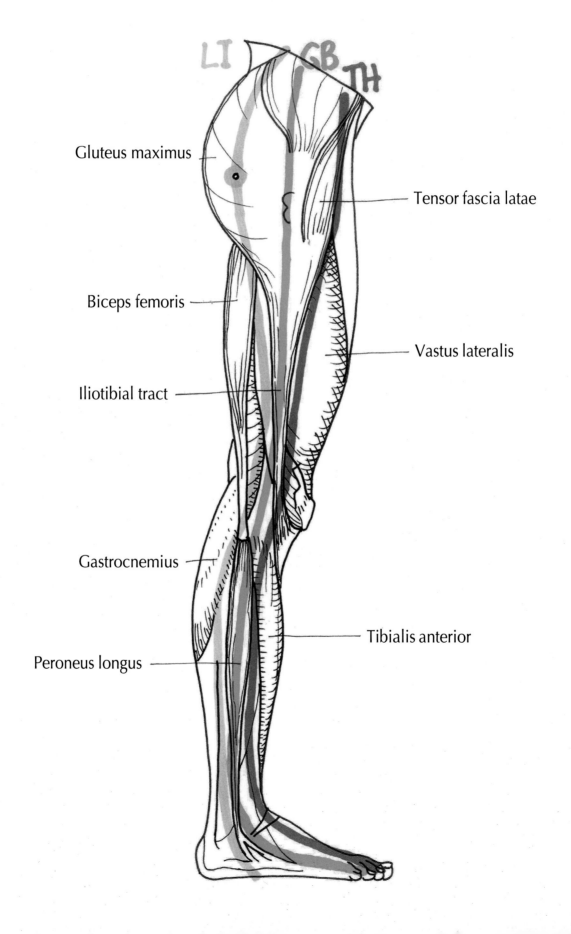

LI   GB   TH

Gluteus maximus

Tensor fascia latae

Biceps femoris

Vastus lateralis

Iliotibial tract

Gastrocnemius

Tibialis anterior

Peroneus longus

12. Posterior Leg All Meridians

On this illustration, traditional KID is coloured dark blue to differentiate from the light blue used for Zen KID.

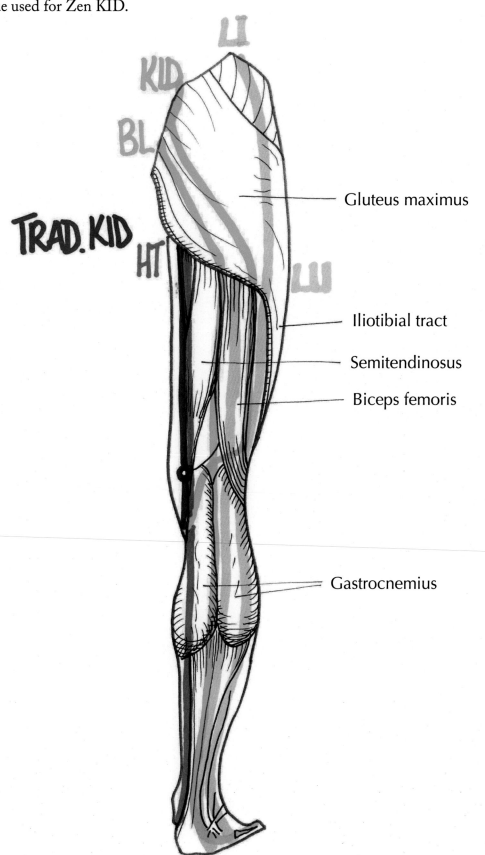

13. Medial Side Leg All Meridians

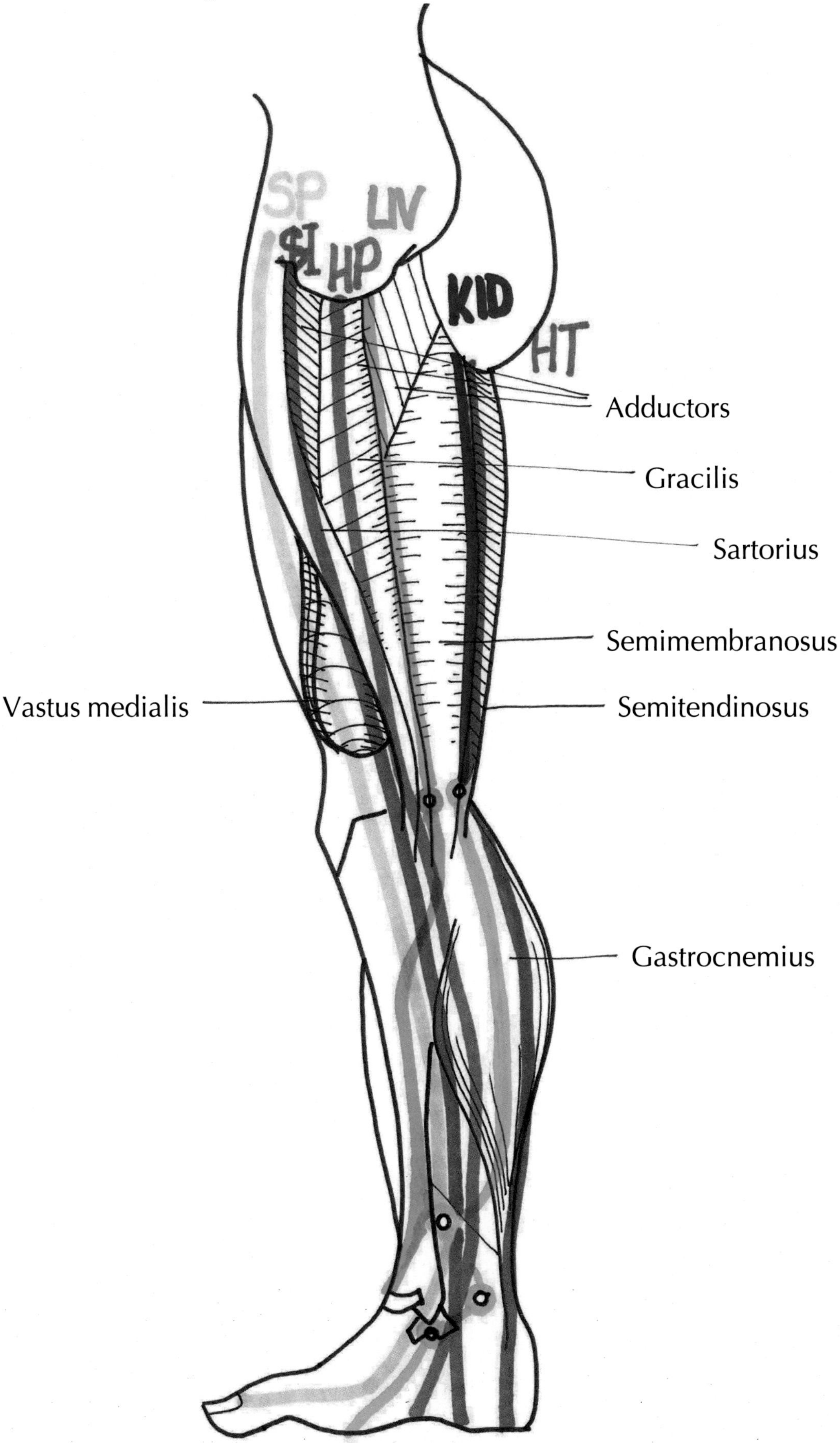

SP
LIV
SI
HP
KID
HT

Adductors

Gracilis

Sartorius

Semimembranosus

Semitendinosus

Vastus medialis

Gastrocnemius

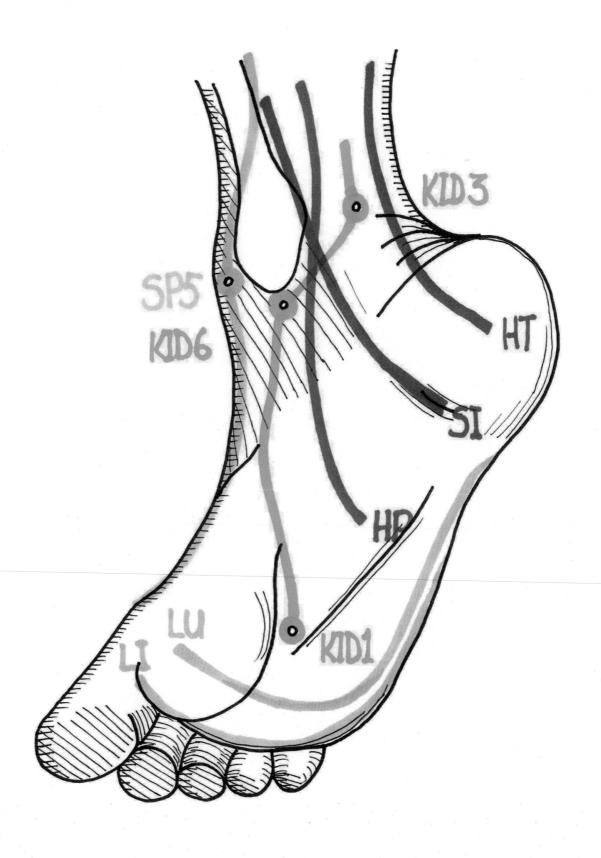

Blank Charts

Blank Torso Anterior

Blank Torso Posterior

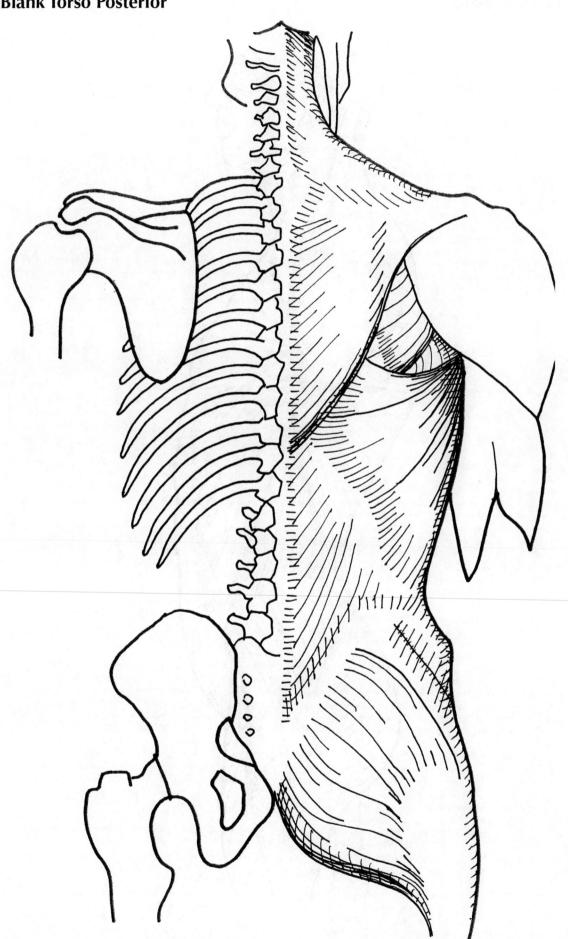

Side View Blank

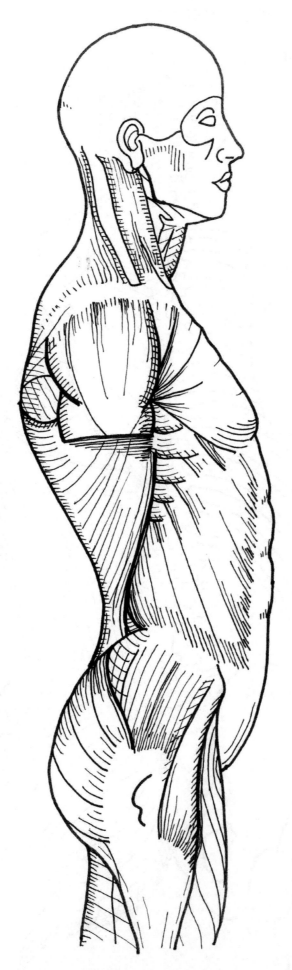

References and Further Reading

References

Deadman, P., Al-Khafaji, M. and Baker, K. (2007) *A Manual of Acupuncture*. Journal of Chinese Medicine.

Beijing College of Traditional Medicine (1980) *Essentials of Chinese Acupuncture*. Beijing: Foreign Languages Press.

Jarmey, C. (2015) The *Concise Book of Muscles*. Chichester: Lotus Publishing.

Masunaga, S. (1970) 'Manual of Diagnosis' unpublished notes, quoted in 'Manual of Diagnosis', *Shiatsu Society News* 103.

Norretranders, T. (1999) *The User Illusion: Cutting Consciousnes Down to Size*. London: Penguin.

Further Reading

Beresford-Cooke, C. (2007) 'Homage to Masunaga', *Shiatsu Society News* 103, p.10.

Beresford-Cooke, C. (2016) *Shiatsu Theory and Practice*. London: Singing Dragon.

Liechti, E. (2002) *Complete Illustrated Guide to Shiatsu*. London: Harper Collins/Element.

Masunaga, S. (1977) *Zen Shiatsu*. Tokyo: Japan Publications.

Rappenecker, W. (2009) *Atlas of Shiatsu*. London: Elsevier Ltd.